Pharmacology and Aphasia

This book provides clinicians and researchers with state-of-the-art research on the pharmacological treatment of aphasia. It focuses on the role of different pharmacological agents to improve aphasia associated with stroke and to attenuate language dissolution in degenerative conditions like Alzheimer's disease and primary progressive aphasia. This book is the first to address these topics.

Leaders in the field provide tutorial reviews on how focal brain injury and degeneration impact on the normal activity of different neurotransmitter systems and how drugs combined or not with rehabilitation can improve language and communication deficits. This is nicely illustrated by studies on single cases and case series describing the beneficial effects of interventions combining drugs with evidence-based rehabilitation techniques. The volume also highlights future directions to refine testing aimed to detect gains in language and non-language cognitive deficits promoted by drug treatment. This book is essential reading for anyone interested in the rehabilitation of aphasia and related cognitive disorders.

This book was originally published as a special issue of *Aphasiology*.

Marcelo L. Berthier is a member of the Unidad de Neurología Cognitiva y Afasia of the Centro de Investigaciones Médico-Sanitarias at the University of Malaga, Spain, and is interested in using different strategies to treat aphasia. Most of his current work concerns the treatment of post-stroke aphasia combining intensive rehabilitation with drugs.

Guadalupe Dávila is a member of the Unidad de Neurología Cognitiva y Afasia of the Centro de Investigaciones Médico-Sanitarias at the University of Malaga, Spain, and is interested in using different strategies to treat aphasia. Most of his current work concerns the treatment of post-stroke aphasia combining intensive rehabilitation with drugs.

Pharmacology and Aphasia

Edited by

Marcelo L. Berthier and Guadalupe Dávila

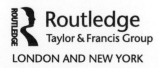

Routledge
Taylor & Francis Group

LONDON AND NEW YORK

First published 2015 by Routledge

2 Park Square, Milton Park, Abingdon, Oxon, OX14 4RN
605 Third Avenue, New York, NY 10017

Routledge is an imprint of the Taylor & Francis Group, an informa business

First issued in paperback 2020

British Library Cataloguing in Publication Data
A catalogue record for this book is available from the British Library

ISBN 13: 978-1-138-79988-2 (hbk)
ISBN 13: 978-0-367-73892-1 (pbk)

Typeset in Times New Roman
by RefineCatch Limited, Bungay, Suffolk

Publisher's Note
The publisher accepts responsibility for any inconsistencies that may have
arisen during the conversion of this book from journal articles to book chapters,
namely the possible inclusion of journal terminology.

Disclaimer
Every effort has been made to contact copyright holders for their permission to
reprint material in this book. The publishers would be grateful to hear from any
copyright holder who is not here acknowledged and will undertake to rectify
any errors or omissions in future editions of this book.

Contents

Contents

Citation Information

The chapters in this book were originally published in *Aphasiology*, volume 23, issue 2 (February 2014). When citing this material, please use the original page numbering for each article, as follows:

Chapter 1
Cognitive enhancing drugs in aphasia: A vote for hope
Marcelo L. Berthier
Aphasiology, volume 23, issue 2 (February 2014) pp. 128–132

Chapter 2
Psycholinguistics of aphasia pharmacotherapy: Asking the right questions
Dalia Cahana-Amitay, Martin L. Albert, and Abigail Oveis
Aphasiology, volume 23, issue 2 (February 2014) pp. 133–154

Chapter 3
Dopaminergic therapy in aphasia
Sumanjit K. Gill and Alexander P. Leff
Aphasiology, volume 23, issue 2 (February 2014) pp. 155–170

Chapter 4
A clinical study of the combined use of bromocriptine and speech and language therapy in the treatment of a person with aphasia
Mandy A. Galling, Neetish Goorah, Marcelo L. Berthier, and Karen Sage
Aphasiology, volume 23, issue 2 (February 2014) pp. 171–187

Chapter 5
Massed sentence repetition training can augment and speed up recovery of speech production deficits in patients with chronic conduction aphasia receiving donepezil treatment
Marcelo L. Berthier, Guadalupe Dávila, Cristina Green-Heredia, Ignacio Moreno Torres, Rocío Juárez y Ruiz de Mier, Irene De-Torres, and Rafael Ruiz-Cruces
Aphasiology, volume 23, issue 2 (February 2014) pp. 188–218

Please direct any queries you may have about the citations to clsuk.permissions@cengage.com

INTRODUCTION

Cognitive enhancing drugs in aphasia: A vote for hope

Marcelo L. Berthier

Unit of Cognitive Neurology and Aphasia, Centro de Investigaciones
Médico-Sanitarias (CIMES), University of Malaga, Malaga, Spain

The effectiveness of aphasia therapy is undisputed, even in patients with long-lasting deficits due to stroke and traumatic brain injury (Basso, Forbes, & Boller, 2013; Cicerone et al., 2011). Benefits are particularly evident when therapies are grounded in neuroscientific principles and when interventions are sufficiently intensive and/or prolonged to promote enduring brain changes in areas participating in recovery. Despite the innovation provided by several groundbreaking interventions (see Basso et al., 2013; Fucetola, Tucker, Blank, & Corbetta, 2005), a research-to-practice gap still exists because the feasibility of delivering optimally effective treatments into everyday clinical practice is limited (Code & Petheram, 2011). To complicate matters further, benefits provided by aphasia therapy are sometimes modest and short-lived and gains do not translate into functional communication. This, coupled with other drawbacks (e.g., aging, mobility problems, limitations imposed by third party insurers), diminish the participation and adherence of patients to aphasia rehabilitation. Therefore, it is imperative to augment and speed up recovery from aphasia through the use of complimentary interventions.

Efforts to integrate insights from cognitive-behavioural models with biological perspectives are providing a growing understanding of the interplay between brain and language in normal and pathological conditions (Husain & Mehta, 2011; Pulvermüller & Berthier, 2008; Varley, 2011). In this context, current efforts are focused on devising successful strategies that boost the gains provided by aphasia therapy. Several augmentative and alternate interventions (drugs, transcranial magnetic and direct current stimulation, speech-generating devices) are currently used to improve language and communication deficits (Cherney et al., 2012; Crinion, 2012; Holland & Crinion, 2012; Small & Llano, 2009). Amongst these, the most widely investigated augmentative approach is the use of drugs. This strategy is known as "cognitive enhancement" (Husain & Mehta, 2011), a term that may be

I would like to thank all contributing authors who have worked hard to comply with tight deadlines, and also to the reviewers of their manuscripts. Also, I would like to thank Professor Chris Code for inviting me to act as the Guest Editor of this Special Issue and the Routledge team.

interchangeable with "neuroreplacement" (Shisler, Baylis, & Frank, 2000), "neuro-modulation" (Floel & Cohen, 2010) and "neuroenhacement" (Repantis, Laisney, & Heuser, 2010).

The rationale for using drugs to ameliorate language deficits in vascular, traumatic and degenerative aphasias is to restore the activity of neurotransmitter systems depleted or released after damage to cortical structure and/or interruption of trans-mitter pathways *en route* from their origins in the brainstem and basal forebrain to deep grey nuclei and cerebral cortex. The effects of drugs on the brain are not limited to a key region; some neurotransmitters (e.g., glutamate) are present in virtually every part of the brain, whereas others (e.g., acetylcholine) innervate more discrete cortical fields. This implies that pharmacological interventions are not targeting exclusively language and communication deficits; rather, the pharmacological mod-ulation of neurotransmitter systems in aphasia is aimed to improve neural efficiency not only in dysfunctional language areas, but also in non-language regions which interact with different language processes through regulation of attention, cognitive control, short-term memory, mood and goal-directed behaviour (motivation).

At present, the activity of several neurotransmitter systems (dopaminergic, choli-nergic, glutamatergic, serotinergic, norepinephrinergic) has been manipulated in aphasia with variable success using agents (levodopa, propranolol, bromocriptine, donepezil, galantamine, memantine) originally marketed to alleviate motor and cognitive-behavioural deficits in Parkinson's disease (PD) and Alzheimer's disease (AD). There is moderate evidence (Level 1b) based on randomised controlled trials ("proof-of-concept" studies) that use of levodopa, donepezil, galantamine and mem-antine may be beneficial in the treatment of chronic vascular aphasia (see Berthier, Pulvermüller, Dávila, Casares, & Gutiérrez, 2011; Salter, Teasell, Bhogal, Zettler, & Foley, 2012; Teasell et al., 2012). It should be noted, however, that none of these drugs is licensed for therapeutic use in aphasia associated to stroke, traumatic brain injury, primary progressive aphasia and other conditions and hence, these agents are prescribed in clinical practice as "off-label" medications. Moreover, the licences of these drugs have recently expired in several countries, thus imposing a limitation to progress in optimising drug treatment of aphasia with these compounds due to the lack of profit incentives to evaluate the efficacy of patent-expired medications.

This special issue of *Aphasiology* is devoted to original studies and reviews addressing the topic of drug treatment of aphasic deficits in patients with focal stroke lesions and degenerative dementias. Cahana-Amitay, Albert, and Oveis (2014) review the mechanisms of aphasia recovery and the different neurotransmitters that can be pharmacologically manipulated to improve language deficits. The authors advocate using a psycholinguistic approach to evaluate language outcomes of pharmacological treatments in aphasia because the usual primary outcome measures (e.g., Western Aphasia Battery) are coarse-grained to identify linguistic deficits amenable to treatment.

Gill and Leff (2014) review the literature on dopaminergic therapy in vascular, traumatic and degenerative aphasias paying particular attention to both the effec-tiveness of the different dopaminergic agents and the cognitive mechanisms modu-lated by dopaminergic drugs underpinning normal and disordered language. Also, they emphasise the need to test the role of new dopaminergic compounds (e.g., rotigotine) to examine whether or not modern drugs provide more benefits and less adverse events than old ones (bromocriptine). Gill and Leff highlight the importance of combining new dopaminergic drugs with neuro-rehabilitation and recommend expanding the assessment of outcome measures to motoric and attentional functions modulated by the dopaminergic system.

In a single case study, Galling, Goorah, Berthier, and Sage (2014) examine the role of combining the dopaminergic agent bromocriptine with aphasia therapy in a stroke patient with chronic nonfluent aphasia and poor engagement in rehabilitation. This study addresses some key points raised by Gill and Leff (2014) and demonstrates that the combined therapy (bromocriptine and aphasia therapy) resulted in greater benefit language and cognitive deficits (attention) and engagement in rehabilitation than either therapy used independently.

In a case series study, Berthier et al. (2014) compare the benefit provided by two therapies (conventional speech language therapy *versus* massed sentence repetition therapy) in three stroke patients with chronic conduction aphasia receiving donepezil treatment. They found that both interventions significantly improved speech production deficits relative to baselines assessments, but outcomes after massed sentence repetition therapy were better than the conventional regime. This paper incorporates some of the recommendations advanced by Cahana-Amitay et al. (2014) regarding the assessment of language functions within the psycholinguistic framework in patients receiving combined treatment with drugs and aphasia therapy.

The last two papers address the issue of pharmacotherapy of degenerative aphasias reviewing the role of several compounds including cholinesterase inhibitors and the NMDA receptor antagonist memantine in language deficits associated with AD. The review paper by Falchook, Heilman, Finney, Gonzalez-Rothi, and Nadeau (2014) focus on the mechanisms of anomia in AD and the role of several compounds, most noticeably donepezil, in improving naming deficits. These authors review their own data showing that the sole utilisation of donepezil provides modest improvements in anomia in comparison with baseline scores, whereas substantial treatment effects can be observed in half of the patients when drug donation was combined with theory-based aphasia rehabilitation (errorless learning). In the other paper, Tocco et al. (2014) review the extant data on the beneficial role of memantine in language and communication deficits among patients with moderate-to-severe AD. Some important results from the reviewed data deserve mention. Patients with moderate-to-severe AD receiving high doses of memantine showed significant less decline in semantic fluency compared with those treated with placebo and the same holds for demented patients with PD. The importance of abnormal communication on the emergence and persistence of psychological and behavioural deficits in AD has been recognised only recently (Saxton et al., 2012) and it seems that memantine treatment in this population provide benefits not only in functional communication, but also in related agitation and aggression.

Although much work need to be done, the studies in this special issue advance our knowledge on the promising role of drug treatment in aphasia and provide some clues for further analysis and intervention. Although the efficacy of drug treatment alone (unpaired with aphasia therapy) requires further analysis, pharmacotherapy should preferentially be administered in combination with tailor-made rehabilitation techniques that promote experience-dependent plasticity. It seems that augmenting the benefits provided by aphasia therapy with drugs can be associated with better outcomes than other strategies and long-term maintenance of benefits, but further studies on the long-term evolution and maintenance of gains after drug withdrawal are warranted. Moreover, it remains to be determined if drugs can improve cognitive domains other than language functions. To test this possibility, potential changes induced by pharmacotherapy in attention, executive function, short-term and episodic memory dependent on the activity of cortical extrasylvian areas should be examined. In the same vein, since aphasia often has a tremendous impact on psychosocial well-being reducing adaptability and return to previous lifestyle, examining the role of cognitive enhancing drugs in alleviating a number of aphasia-related complications (depression, stress, anxiety, apathy, hopelessness and social isolation) is of paramount importance.

REFERENCES

Basso, A., Forbes, M., & Boller, F. (2013). Rehabilitation of aphasia. *Handbook of Clinical Neurology, 110*, 325–334. doi:10.1016/B978-0-444-52901-5.00027-7

Berthier, M. L., Dávila, G., Green, C., Moreno-Torres, I., Juárez y Ruiz de Mier, R., De-Torres, I, & Ruiz-Cruces, R. (2014). Massed sentence repetition training can augment and speed up recovery of speech production deficits in patients with chronic conduction aphasia receiving donepezil treatment. *Aphasiology, 28*, 188–218.

Berthier, M. L., Pulvermüller, F., Dávila, G., Casares, N., & Gutiérrez, A. (2011). Drug therapy of post-stroke aphasia: A review of current evidence. *Neuropsychology Review, 21*, 302–317. doi:10.1007/s11065-011-9177-7

Cahana-Amitay, D., Albert, M. L., & Oveis, A. (2014). Psycholinguistics of aphasia pharmacotherapy: Asking the right questions. *Aphasiology, 28*, 133–154.

Cherney, L. R., Harvey, R. L., Babbitt, E. M., Hurwitz, R., Kaye, R. C., Lee, J. B., ... Small, S. L. (2012). Epidural cortical stimulation and aphasia therapy. *Aphasiology, 26*, 1192–1217. doi:10.1080/02687038.2011.603719

Cicerone, K. D., Langenbahn, D. M., Braden, C., Malec, J. F., Kalmar, K., Fraas, M., ... Ashman, T. (2011). Evidence-based cognitive rehabilitation: Updated review of the literature from 2003 through 2008. *Archives of Physical Medicine and Rehabilitation, 92*, 519–530. doi:10.1016/j.apmr.2010.11.015

Code, C., & Petheram, B. (2011). Delivering for aphasia. *International Journal of Speech and Language Pathology, 13*, 3–10. doi:10.3109/17549507.2010.520090

Crinion, J. (2012). Shocking speech. *Aphasiology, 26*, 1077–1081. doi:10.1080/02687038.2012.714215

Falchook, A. D., Heilman, K. M., Finney, G. R., Gonzalez-Rothi, L. J., & Nadeau, S. E. (2014). Neuroplasticity, neurotransmitters, and new directions for treatment of anomia in Alzheimer disease. *Aphasiology, 28*, 219–235.

Floel, A., & Cohen, L. G. (2010). Recovery of function in humans: Cortical stimulation and pharmacological treatments after stroke. *Neurobiology of Disease, 37*, 243–251. doi:10.1016/j.nbd.2009.05.027

Fucetola, R., Tucker, F., Blank, K., & Corbetta, M. (2005). A process for translating evidence-based aphasia treatment into clinical practice. *Aphasiology, 19*, 411–422. doi:10.1080/02687030444000859

Galling, M. A., Goorah, N., Berthier, M. L., & Sage, K. (2014). A clinical study of the combined use of bromocriptine and speech and language therapy in the treatment of a person with aphasia. *Aphasiology, 28*, 171–187.

Gill, S. K., & Leff, A. (2014). Dopaminergic therapy in aphasia. *Aphasiology, 28*, 155–170.

Holland, R., & Crinion, J. (2012). Can tDCS enhance treatment of aphasia after stroke? *Aphasiology, 26*, 1169–1191. doi:10.1080/02687038.2011.616925

Husain, M., & Mehta, M. A. (2011). Cognitive enhancement by drugs in health and disease. *Trends in Cognitive Sciences, 15*, 28–36. doi:10.1016/j.tics.2010.11.002

Pulvermüller, F., & Berthier, M. L. (2008). Aphasia therapy on a neuroscience basis. *Aphasiology, 22*, 563–599. doi:10.1080/02687030701612213

Repantis, D., Laisney, O., & Heuser, I. (2010). Acetylcholinesterase inhibitors and memantine for neuroenhancement in healthy individuals: A systematic review. *Pharmacological Research, 61*, 473–481. doi:10.1016/j.phrs.2010.02.009

Salter, K., Teasell, R., Bhogal, S., Zettler, L., & Foley, N. (2012). *The evidence-based review of stroke rehabilitation (EBRSR) reviews current practices in stroke rehabilitation.* (Chapter 14: Aphasia). Retrieved from http:\\www.ebrsr.com.

Saxton, J., Hofbauer, R. K., Woodward, M., Gilchrist, N. L., Potocnik, F., & Hsu, H. A. (2012). Memantine and functional communication in Alzheimer's disease: Results of a 12-week, international, randomized clinical trial. *Journal of Alzheimer's Disease, 28*, 109–118.

Shisler, R. J., Baylis, G. C., & Frank, E. M. (2000). Pharmacological approaches to the treatment and prevention of aphasia. *Aphasiology, 14*, 1163–1186. doi:10.1080/02687030050205705

Small, S. L., & Llano, D. A. (2009). Biological approaches to aphasia treatment. *Current Neurology and Neuroscience Reports, 9*, 443–450. doi:10.1007/s11910-009-0066-x

Teasell, R., Foley, N., Salter, K., Bhogal, S., Jutai, J., & Speechley, M. (2012). *Evidence-based review of stroke rehabilitation. Executive summary* (15th ed.). Retrieved from http:\\www.ebrsr.com

Tocco, M., Bayles, K., Lopez, O. L., Hofbauer, R. K., Pejović, V., Miller, M. L., ... Saxton, J. (2014). Effects of memantine treatment on language abilities and functional communication: A review of data. *Aphasiology, 28*, 236–257.

Varley, R. (2011). Rethinking aphasia therapy: A neuroscience perspective. *International Journal of Speech-Language Pathology, 13*, 11–20. doi:10.3109/17549507.2010.497561

Psycholinguistics of aphasia pharmacotherapy: Asking the right questions

Dalia Cahana-Amitay, Martin L. Albert, and Abigail Oveis

Department of Neurology, Harold Goodglass Aphasia Research Center, VA Boston Healthcare System, Boston University School of Medicine, Boston, MA, USA

Background: Among the obstacles to demonstrating efficacy of pharmacological intervention for aphasia is quantifying patients' responses to treatment in a statistically valid and reliable manner. In many of the review papers on this topic, detailed discussions of various methodological problems are highlighted, with some suggestions on how these shortcomings should be addressed. Given this deep understanding of caveats associated with the experimental design of aphasia pharmacotherapy studies, investigations continue to produce inconsistent results.

Aim: In this review paper, we suggest that the inclusion of theory-driven linguistic measures in aphasia pharmacotherapy studies would add an important step toward elucidating precise patterns of improvement in language performance resulting from pharmacotherapeutic intervention.

Main Contribution: We provide a brief review of the clinical approaches currently used in pharmacotherapy studies of aphasia, which often lack psycholinguistic grounding. We then present ways in which psycholinguistic models can complement this approach, offering a rationale for task selection, and as a result, lead to a better understanding of treatment effects. We then follow with an example of how such an integrative approach can be implemented in studies targeting stress reduction in people with aphasia, via beta-blocking agents, as a means to augment language performance, using the recently proposed psycholinguistic framework of "linguistic anxiety" as our guideline.

Conclusion: We conclude that the incorporation of psycholinguistic models into aphasia pharmacotherapy studies can increase the resolution with which we can identify functional changes.

We thank Emmanuel Ojo for his contribution to the preparation of this manuscript. We also thank Ron Spiro and our anonymous reviewers for their insightful comments. Support for this research was provided by the National Institutes of Health, NIDCD grant 5P30DC005207 and NIA grant 2R01AG14345, Boston University School of Medicine, Department of Neurology, Harold Goodglass Aphasia Research Center and VA Boston Healthcare System, 150 South Huntington Avenue, Boston, MA 02130.

Over the past quarter century, pharmacotherapy has been recognised as a potential adjunct to other therapeutic approaches for treatment of language impairment due to brain damage (e.g., Albert, 1988; Berthier et al., 2011; Beversdorf, Narayanan, Hillier, & Hughes, 2007; De Boissezon, Peran, De Boysson, & Démonet, 2007; Klein & Albert, 2004; McNamara & Albert, 2004; Mimura, Albert, & McNamara, 1995; Small, 1994, 2000; Small & Llano, 2009). Research efforts addressing the efficacy of such interventions have largely been guided by a clinical approach, with loose reference to neurobiology, whereby post-stroke neurochemical abnormalities are implicated in the breakdown of particular cognitive systems, and so can serve as targets of therapy. This approach is rooted in studies demonstrating how neurochemical manipulations of noradrenergic, dopaminergic, cholinergic and glutamatergic mechanisms restore brain function in animal and human models (e.g., Small & Llano, 2009). However, in spite of encouraging results and the enthusiasm of its proponents, empirical findings describing beneficial effects of pharmacotherapy on language disorders remain limited, with mixed reports that call into question the efficacy of such treatments (e.g., Berthier et al., 2011; De Boissezon et al., 2007). It should come as no surprise, then, that "a language enhancement pill" has yet to find its way into common clinical practice in the treatment of language impairment. (For other factors limiting consistent use of drugs in aphasia treatment, see Berthier et al., 2011.)

What is it that makes results from pharmacotherapy studies of language impairment so elusive? Many of the observed inconsistencies are anchored in methodological problems (Berthier et al., 2011; De Boissezon et al., 2007; Small & Llano, 2009). These include issues such as sample selection (ignoring mixed aetiologies as a source of variability in responsiveness to drug treatment), sample size (questioning the value of findings from case studies, small sample studies), time post-onset (difficulty differentiating effects of spontaneous recovery from those of drug treatment), study design (bias in open label studies vs. randomised double-blind controlled trial, randomised double-blind placebo-controlled trial, randomised examiner-blind clinical trial), dosage of drugs administered (overdosing having the potential of leading to neurochemical dysregulation, worsening treatment outcomes), duration of intervention (interventions being insufficiently long to bring about change) and administration of drugs with concomitant language therapies (reduced efficacy of drugs as stand-alone treatments).

In this paper, we suggest an additional step in experimental design that may bring us closer to the goal of quantifying patient outcomes with increased precision. Specifically, we suggest that in the absence of theory-driven linguistic measures, it would be difficult to elucidate precise patterns of improvement in language performance resulting from pharmacotherapeutic intervention. Such a view has also been voiced by (Rapp, Caplan, Edwards, Visch-Brink, & Thompson, 2013), who pointed out the importance of task selection for interpretation of treatment effects in neuroimaging studies. We thus propose an integrative approach to the study of pharmacotherapy of language disorders: neurobiological considerations in selection of pharmacologic agents should be combined with theory-driven psycholinguistic considerations. This integrative approach might thereby allow researchers to pose confirmable hypotheses that could shed *new* light on the potential neurochemical systems correlated with specific linguistic deficits, leading to more precisely targeted interventions.

Our intention here is not to review once again the neurobiological promise that pharmacotherapy of aphasia may hold, but rather to highlight the importance of integrating psycholinguistic considerations into the design of such studies, which are essential for understanding the effects of such treatment. In what follows, then, we provide a brief review of the clinical approaches currently used in pharmacotherapy studies of aphasia, which have often been based on classical aphasiological phenomenology and, often, lack psycholinguistic grounding. We then present ways in which psycholinguistic models can complement this approach, offering a rationale for task selection, and as a result, lead to a better understanding of treatment effects. We then follow with an example of how such an integrative approach can be implemented in studies targeting stress reduction as a means to augment language performance in people with aphasia (see also Cahana-Amitay et al., 2011). Our focus in this review will primarily be on post-stroke aphasia, although pharmacotherapy studies for language disorders are also being conducted in patients with other neurologic conditions, such as Parkinson's disease and primary progressive aphasia (see, for example, Angwin, Copland, Chenery, Murdoch, & Silburn, 2006; Reed, Johnson, Thompson, Weintraub, & Mesulam, 2004).

PHARMACOTHERAPY OF APHASIA: CURRENT PERSPECTIVES

Pharmacotherapy is one of the several biological approaches to the treatment of aphasia used to stimulate post-stroke neural reorganisation, on the premise that observed functional recovery directly reflects reparation of neural circuits mediating language and other cognitive functions (e.g., Lee & Hillis, 2008; Small & Llano, 2009).

MECHANISMS OF APHASIA RECOVERY: RATIONALE

Neurochemical interventions for aphasia are designed, among other reasons, to strengthen networks subserving language and language-related cognitive functions such as attention and memory (e.g., Berthier & Pulvermüller, 2011; Floel & Cohen, 2010). As previously pointed out, " . . . no single neurotransmitter is likely to underlie any complex cognitive process. Most such processes likely depend on the dynamic interplay of many neuromodulators, some perhaps not even identified as yet . . . " (Albert, 2000, p. 157). Broadly speaking, recovery of these networks is associated with activation or re-activation of brain tissue in both the right and left hemispheres (e.g., Klein & Albert, 2004), which is accomplished via "reactive plasticity" (e.g., Nadeau & Wu, 2006). At the cellular level, different mechanisms are assumed to be involved in this process, e.g., neurogenesis, cell migration, axonal sprouting, dendritic elaboration and changes in the excitability of existing synaptic connections. These mechanisms make unique temporal and spatial contributions to the restoration of activity in neural networks, both influenced by and influencing the local and wide-spread consequences of stroke-related factors, including lesion location/size (Heiss & Thiel, 2006; Lazar & Antoniello, 2008), aetiology (Klein & Albert, 2004), inhibitory and excitatory effects of various pharmacologic agents and therefore are likely to show distinct responses to pharmacotherapeutic interventions (Small & Llano, 2009).

TARGETING NEUROTRANSMITTERS

Neurochemical manipulations of neurotransmitter systems and their effects on language performance in aphasia have been explored in more than forty pharmacotherapy studies (see Berthier et al., 2011; Small & Llano, 2009). These studies examined the efficacy of drugs acting on noradrenergic, dopaminergic, cholinergic and glutamatergic systems. Most efforts have been directed at exploring dopaminergic, noradrenergic and cholinergic effects, primarily on naming. The research focus in these studies was never driven by an explicit theory of "neurochemistry of language," but speculations were made about ways in which pharmacosystems might mediate certain aspects of lexical retrieval. Albert (2000), for example, proposed that dopaminergic pathways might support, in part, phonological output and articulation, whereas cholinergic pathways might contribute to lexical semantics. Beversdorf et al. (2007) considered the role of reducing noradrenergic activity to suppress background neural activation, to increase the efficiency of lexical-semantic searches among people with aphasia with intact error monitoring (Beversdorf et al., 2007).

DOPAMINERGIC AND NORADRENERGIC SYSTEMS: CATECHOLAMINES

The most widely investigated class of drugs so far has been the catecholamines (e.g., Albert, 1988; Arciniegas, Frey, Anderson, Brousseau, & Harris, 2004; Berthier, 2005, 2009; De Boissezon et al., 2007; Leeman, Laganaro, Chetelat-Mabillard, & Schnider, 2011; McNeil et al., 1997; Raymer, 2003; Raymer et al., 2001; Walker-Batson et al., 1992, 2001; Whiting, Chenery, Chalk, & Copland, 2007), such as Bromocriptine, Levodopa, Dextroamphetamine and Amantadine, which are involved in neuromodulation of the dopaminergic and noradrenergic systems. Many of these pharmacotherapeutic interventions were carried out on the assumption that drugs targeting dopaminergic and noradrenergic deficiencies in damaged prefrontal, motor and association cortices could improve language and speech motor functions associated with these areas, such as impaired lexical retrieval and verbal perseveration (e.g., Albert, 2000; McNamara & Albert, 2004). It was thought, for example, that stimulation of these neurotransmitter systems could benefit people with aphasia by augmenting the attentional systems necessary for activating different language output systems (Alexander, 2006; Crosson et al., 2005).

The expectation that language output would be positively affected by such neurochemical manipulation was supported both by evidence showing that the dopaminergic system operates in a lateralised fashion (McNamara & Albert, 2004) and by findings indicating that some catecholaminergic drugs specifically potentiate activity in frontal language-related networks if administered in conjunction with certain language tasks, such as verb generation (Sommer et al., 2006), or artificial vocabulary training (Breitenstein et al., 2004). Long-term retention of novel word learning has also been observed, following the administration of levodopa (Knecht et al., 2004). And, indeed, catecholamines have been shown primarily to affect the disorders of *language output,* with the most efficacious results observed among people with non-fluent aphasia (Klein & Albert, 2004). Administration of dopamine agonists to such patients has been found to enhance speech initiation, reduce pauses and paraphasias in conversations, increase naming accuracy, improve repetition abilities, promote verbal (phonological) fluency and shorten verbal latencies (Albert, 1988; Berthier, 1999, 2005; Bragoni et al., 2000; Raymer, 2003; Raymer et al., 2001; Seniów, Litwin, Litwin, Leśniak, & Członkowska, 2009).

However, these pharmacotherapeutic interventions have shown only varying degrees of success (e.g., Ashtary, Janghorbani, Chitsaz, Reisi, & Bahrami, 2006; Gupta & Mlcoch, 1992; Leeman et al., 2011; Sabe, Salvarezza, García Cuerva, Leiguarda, & Starkstein, 1995). The language gains reported were partial, especially among patients with moderate to severe impairment, in whom certain language problems (e.g., non-fluency) persisted even after treatment, showing limited to no long-term effects (Berthier et al., 2011). These disappointing results are attributable, in part, to one or more of the methodological issues listed in the Introduction. Nonetheless, better efficacy has been reported in studies in which drug delivery was coupled with evidence-based language treatments (e.g., constraint-induced language therapy), where neuroplasticity was enhanced in behaviourally stimulated neural networks (see also Lee & Hillis, 2008; Shisler, Baylis, & Frank, 2000).

CHOLINERGIC- AND GLUTAMATERGIC-BASED DRUGS

Efforts have also been made to investigate the efficacy of drugs targeting cholinergic and glutamatergic neurotransmitter systems for aphasia recovery, such as Ameridin, Bifemelane, Aniracetam, Galantamine, Piracetam, Donepezil and Memantine, inspired, in part, by pharmacotherapy studies in Alzheimer's disease and vascular dementia (Berthier et al., 2011; Klein & Albert, 2004; Small & Llano, 2009). Evidence of increased left-lateralised cholinergic activity in the brain, especially in the temporal lobe (Albert, 2000), has led to the conjecture that a deficiency in this neurotransmitter system might result in adverse effects for language abilities dependent on verbal memory (e.g., Klein & Albert, 2004; Mimura et al., 1995). Patterns of impaired naming and reduced verbal fluency among healthy young women following administration of a drug blocking cholinergic activity (Aarsland, Larsen, Reinvang, & Aasland, 1994) lend support to this idea. Additional support comes from studies reporting perseverative and paraphasic errors among aphasic patients with cholinergic deficiencies (Berthier, Hinojosa, & Moreno-Torre, 2004; Corbett, Jefferies, & Lambon Ralph, 2008; Gotts, Della Rocchetta, & Cipolotti, 2002; McNamara & Albert, 2004).

The mechanisms by which cholinergic- and glutamatergic-based interventions could lead to improved language functions, however, remain unclear. Berthier and colleagues, for example, have suggested that stimulating interrupted cholinergic pathways in damaged basal forebrain, peri-sylvian, brainstem and thalamic areas, can enable encoding of linguistic information and filtering of task-irrelevant noise via top-down increases in sensory input (Berthier & Pulvermüller, 2011; Berthier et al., 2011). This idea is based, in part, on the observation that cholinergic activity is involved in long-term neural potentiation required for processes of attention and learning/memory (Sarter, Hasselmo, Bruno, & Givens, 2005). Stimulation of glutamatergic activity in the brain, in contrast, has been argued to increase the efficiency with which spared neural networks operate, augmenting recovery, especially when coupled with behavioural programs, such as constraint-induced language therapy (Berthier et al., 2009; Pulvermüller et al., 2001).

In several studies, cholinergic or glutamatergic-based interventions have, indeed, been found to improve performance on naming and comprehension tasks among aphasic patients with posterior lesions and patients with fluent aphasia (e.g., Berthier, Hinojosa, Martín, & Fernández, 2003; Berthier et al., 2006, 2009; Chen et al., 2010; Huber, Willmes, Poeck, Van Vleymen, & Deberdt, 1997; Kessler, Thiel, Karbe, & Heiss, 2000; Luriiâ, 1970; Pulvermüller et al., 2001; Tanaka & Albert, 2001; Tanaka, Miyazaki, & Albert, 1997). Language improvements in these studies cover multiple domains, including, for example, improved articulation, increased amount of spontaneous speech, greater naming accuracy, faster latencies, improved repetition, better semantic and phonemic discrimination and enhanced word- and sentence-picture matching abilities (Berthier et al., 2011). In some cases, such improvements have also been associated with increased blood flow in frontotemporal regions (Kessler et al., 2000). Because the most consistent benefits have been observed in word retrieval abilities, and because anomia continues to constitute the hallmark of aphasic language disorder in all patients with long-term aphasia (see Lazar & Antoniello, 2008), drugs, such as donepezil have been argued to be particularly promising for aphasia treatment in its chronic stages (Berthier et al., 2011). However, at this point, claims about the efficacy of these interventions are tentative, as consistent findings of long-term benefits in cases of large lesions are yet to be reported (e.g., Güngör, Terzi, & Onar, 2011).

EFFICACY OF APHASIA PHARMACOTHERAPY: QUANTIFYING EFFECTS

Among the obstacles to demonstrating efficacy of pharmacological intervention for aphasia is quantification of patients' responses to treatment in a statistically valid and reliable manner. No less important is the personal response of the patient. In pharmacotherapy studies of aphasia (or any therapy study, for that matter) statistical improvement on a standardised test must be coupled with a clinically meaningful response. The patient should get better, and know it. In many of the review papers on this topic (e.g., Berthier et al., 2011; De Boissezon et al., 2007; Small & Llano, 2009), detailed discussions of methodological and measurement problems are highlighted, with some suggestions on how shortcomings might be addressed. Small and Llano (2009), for example, stated: "In our view, the optimum study design to establish that a pharmacological agent promotes brain reorganization to enhance language processing would be a double-blind, placebo-controlled, adequately-powered, parallel group study that contains at least one outcome measure that is assessed after drug washout to ensure that any benefit observed is not only due to temporary enhancement of arousal" (p. 445). Berthier et al. (2011) have even conducted a reanalysis of previously collected data (Berthier et al., 2003, 2006) to address the issue of interpatient variability often observed in biological intervention studies (Berthier et al., 2009; Cherney, Erickson, & Small, 2010). They quantified the proportion of participants who responded to the administration of donepezil, a cholinergic-based drug, using changes in Aphasia Quotient scores of the Western Aphasia Battery (Kertesz, Sheppard, & MacKenzie, 1982), compared to baseline performance, as a measure of reduction in aphasia severity.

However, in spite of this deep understanding of the caveats associated with the experimental design of aphasia pharmacotherapy studies (e.g.,Berthier et al., 2011), investigations continue to produce inconsistent results. We believe that this picture is partially determined by the inadequacy of the linguistic measures used in these studies to assess language improvement in treated patients. Selection of relevant diagnostic language tasks in any treatment study should ideally be driven by a theory of language that outlines a certain degree of linguistic specificity, in order to predict where linguistic dysfunction might occur and what kinds of errors can be expected (see Rapp et al., 2013, for an analogous argument). A quick look at the linguistic measures used in many of the published aphasia pharmacotherapy studies indicates that their choice has rarely been motivated by systematic psycholinguistic considerations. Table 1 lists linguistic tasks which have been used to assess treatment-based language change in different aphasia pharmacotherapy studies to date.

TABLE 1

Pre- and post-treatment linguistic measures used in aphasia pharmacotherapy studies

Author, year	Drug	N	Aetiology	Aphasia type & severity (pre-treatment)	Concurrent treatment	Linguistic outcome measures (pre- & post-treatment)	Results
Albert (1988)	Bromocriptine	1	CVA (haemorrhage)	Moderate TCMA; BDAE: 3.5	None specified	BDAE subtests, Cookie Theft picture description, latency of response, pauses	Improvement: reduced latency of response, decreased paraphasias, increased naming ability; language returned to baseline after treatment stopped
MacLennan, Nicholas, Morley, and Brookshire (1991)	Bromocriptine	1	CVA (ischemic)	TCMA	None specified	Captain's Log Stimulus Visual Reaction Time, Token Test, BNT, verbal fluency, BDAE, other speech samples, mood & ability to communicate questionnaire	No significant effect
Gupta and Mlcoch (1992)	Bromocriptine	2	CVA	Non-fluent aphasia	None specified	BDAE, BNT, Mean length of utterance (MLU)	Improvements in verbal fluency and naming; increased MLU
Sabe, Leiguarda, and Starkstein (1992)	Bromocriptine	7	CVA	Moderate to severe non-fluent aphasia; 4 TCMA, 2 Broca's, 1 Global	None specified	WAB figure description: lexical index, grammatical index, verbal fluency, significant words, pauses (>3s)	No improvements for patients with severe aphasia; improvements in lexical index and fluency and decreased number of pauses for the mild patients; these improvements declined after reducing/discontinuing the medication.

(Continued)

TABLE 1
(Continued)

Author, year	Drug	N	Aetiology	Aphasia type & severity (pre-treatment)	Concurrent treatment	Linguistic outcome measures (pre- & post-treatment)	Results
Gupta, Mlcoch, Scolaro, and Moritz (1995)	Bromocriptine	20	Brain injury, unspecified	Non-fluent aphasia; TCMA, Broca's, Mixed	None specified	WAB, BNT, RCPM	No significant effect
Ozeren, Sarica, Mavi, and Demirkiran (1995)	Bromocriptine	4	CVA	Non-fluent aphasia; 2 Broca's, 1 Global, 1 TCMA	None specified	"Aphasia tests"	No effect
Sabe et al. (1995)	Bromocriptine	7	5 CVA (ischemic), 2 TBI	Moderate non-fluent aphasia; 2 Broca's, 3 TCMA, 2 Anomic	None specified	WAB, BDAE figure description, BNT, verbal fluency (FAS)	No significant effect
Gold, Van Dam, and Silliman (2000)	Bromocriptine	4	CVA	Non-fluent Aphasia; 2 Broca's, 2 TCMA; AQ Range: 41–84.8	None specified	Gold, Rosen & Silliman object-naming task; reaction times, storage & retrieval quotients	Improvements in word retrieval quotient; declines in time latency; no effect on word storage quotient
Bragoni et al. (2000)	Bromocriptine	11	CVA	Non-fluent; Broca's, Global; Severity range: mild to severe	Speech therapy, not detailed	Standardised Italian language test; Token test, FAS, set test, sentence generation, visual naming, verbal latency	Improvement observed in dictation, reading comprehension, and verbal latency
Raymer et al. (2001)	Bromocriptine	1	CVA	Crossed non-fluent aphasia; TCMA; WAB Aphasia Quotient: 79.8	None specified	WAB, BNT, verbal fluency (FAS), Florida Apraxia Screening Test-Revised, procedural discourse	Improvement in verbal fluency; no improvement in gesture or emotional prosody
Reed et al. (2004)	Bromocriptine	6	Progressive	PPA	None specified	Discourse analysis: MLU, proportion of grammatical sentences, noun-verb ratio, open-class/closed-class	No significant effect

(Continued)

TABLE 1
(Continued)

Author, year	Drug	N	Aetiology	Aphasia type & severity (pre-treatment)	Concurrent treatment	Linguistic outcome measures (pre- & post-treatment)	Results
Ashtary et al. (2006)	Bromocriptine	38	CVA	Non-fluent aphasia	None specified	Standardised Persian language test	No significant effect
Seniow et al. (2009)	Levodopa	39	CVA	All levels of aphasia severity range (0–5)	SLT: 45 minutes, 5 days/week for 3 weeks	BDAE	Language improvements in verbal fluency and repetition, particularly among patients with anterior lesions
Leeman et al. (2011)	Levodopa	12	CVA, TBI	Wernicke's, Broca's, Conduction, Anomia	SLT: standard clinical treatment (4–5 hrs/week); additional daily Computerised Aphasia Therapy (CAT)	Battery of naming tasks	No significant effect
Walker-Batson et al. (1992)	D-amphetamine	1	CVA	Broca-type aphasia; AQ: 32.5	SLT: 75 minutes every 4th day for 6 weeks (12.5 hours); treatment focused on verbal performance	PICA, BDAE	PICA improvement greater than PICA recovery prediction
McNeil, Small, Masterson, and Fossett (1995)	D-amphetamine	1	Progressive	PPA	SLT: Individual sessions 3 hrs/week for 5 months; focused on cuing hierarchy for producing antonym and synonym adjectives	PICA, Revised Token Test, RCPM, RAN, standardised narrative discourse	Treatment effective for antonym and synonym adjectives; language declines in standardised domains; differential effects of behavioural treatment and pharmacological + behavioural intervention were not observed

(Continued)

TABLE 1
(Continued)

Author, year	Drug	N	Aetiology	Aphasia type & severity (pre-treatment)	Concurrent treatment	Linguistic outcome measures (pre- & post-treatment)	Results
McNeil et al. (1997)	D-amphetamine	2	CVA	Mild to moderate aphasia and co-occurring apraxia of speech	Lexical-semantic activation inhibition therapy (L-SAIT) present in one condition, absent in one condition	RAN, connected speech measures	No effects in absence of L-SAIT; positive treatment effects attributed to L-SAIT
Walker-Batson et al. (2001)	D-amphetamine	21	Non-haemorrhagic infarction	Aphasia, PICA score between 10–70	SLT: 1-hr individual session 3–4 days/week; protocol individualised as needed for each patient's specific needs	PICA	D-amphetamine paired with speech/language treatment accelerated rate of recovery in sub-acute stage
Whiting et al. (2007)	D-amphetamine	2		Chronic aphasia	SLT: 2, 4-week blocks of naming therapy, 2–3 sessions/week	Confrontation naming task	Greater therapy progress with addition of d-amphetamine rather than placebo; improvement difference significant for only one individual
Darley, Keith, and Sasanuma (1977)	Methylphenidate vs. chlordiazepoxide	14	TBI, CVA		None specified	PICA, Word fluency	No effect of either drug
Barrett and Eslinger (2007)	Amantadine	4	CVA, CVA + aneurysm surgery, brain tumour resection	Non-fluent; TCMA	SLT: 1 hr, 5 days/week	Controlled Oral Word Association Test	Improvements in word generation

(Continued)

TABLE 1
(Continued)

Author, year	Drug	N	Aetiology	Aphasia type & severity (pre-treatment)	Concurrent treatment	Linguistic outcome measures (pre- & post-treatment)	Results
Kertesz et al. (2008)	Galantamine	36	Progressive	PPA	None specified	Frontal Behaviour Inventory, WAB, Clinical Global Impression of Severity, Clinical Global Impression of Improvement	No significant differences in behaviour or language; language scores for galantamine group remained stable while placebo group scores deteriorated
Hong, Shin, Lim, Lee, and Huh (2012)	Galantamine	45	CVA	Chronic aphasia	None specified	Four domains of WAB-AQ; MMSE	Significant increase in AQ scores for galantamine group but not control group
Tanaka et al. (1997)	Bifemelane	4	CVA	Fluent aphasia	SLT: conventional aphasia therapy 3 times/week	Standard Language Test for Aphasia	Improvements in comprehension and naming for treatment group; no change in language for non-treatment group
Tanaka and Albert (2001)	Aniracetam	8	CVA	Wernicke's aphasia, mild and severe	None specified	BNT, ANT, Word generation test for categories, tests of perseveration; tests of verbal memory	Improvement on BNT, ANT, word generation and decreased perseveration for non-severe patients
Pashek and Bachman (2003)	Donepezil	1	CVA	Broca's aphasia with moderately severe verbal apraxia	None specified	BNT, ANT, BDAE, Token test, attention tests	Consistent improvement in language, cognition and motor speech; improvements maintained at follow-up testing

(Continued)

TABLE 1
(Continued)

Author, year	Drug	N	Aetiology	Aphasia type & severity (pre-treatment)	Concurrent treatment	Linguistic outcome measures (pre- & post-treatment)	Results
Berthier et al. (2006)	Donepezil	26	CVA	Broca's, anomic, conduction, and Wernicke's aphasia	SLT: 2 hrs/week; Syndrome-specific standard approach	WAB, CAL, PALPA, Stroke Aphasic Depression Questionnaire	Improvement in aphasia severity with donepezil relative to placebo
Chen et al. (2010)	Donepezil	60	CVA	Acute aphasia	None specified	WAB	Significantly greater improvement in donepezil group than control group
Berthier et al. (2009)	Memantine	27	CVA (ischemic, haemorrhagic)	Chronic aphasia	CIAT; 30 hours within 2 weeks for each patient	WAB, CAL	Greater improvement with CIAT and memantine treatment than CIAT alone; beneficial effects persisted long-term
Johnson et al. (2010)	Memantine	18	Progressive	Mild to moderate PPA	None specified	WAB	No significant effect; smaller degree of decline on WAB aphasia quotient in drug group
Huber et al. (1997)	Piracetam	66	CVA, TBI, brain surgery unrelated to malignant tumour	Moderate to severe aphasia	Speech Therapy: 10 (5 individual, 5 group) sessions; 60-min sessions/week for 6 weeks	AAT	Greater significance for piracetam than placebo for "written language" and "profile level"
Orgogozo (1999)	Piracetam	373	CVA (ischemic)		SLT, not detailed	Frenchay Aphasia Screening Test	Greater percentage with aphasia recovery in piracetam group compared to placebo group

(Continued)

TABLE 1
(Continued)

Author, year	Drug	N	Aetiology	Aphasia type & severity (pre-treatment)	Concurrent treatment	Linguistic outcome measures (pre- & post-treatment)	Results
Kessler et al. (2000)	Piracetam	24	CVA (ischemic)	Mild to moderate aphasia	SLT: 5 60-min sessions/week for 6 weeks	AAT, FAS, Corsi's block span test, tests of apraxia, RCPM, Benton Test	AAT: piracetam increased 7 sub-scores
Gungor et al. (2011)	Piracetam	30	CVA (ischemic)	moderate to severe aphasia	None specified	NIHSS, Gulhane Aphasia Test	No clear benefit
Tanaka, Albert, Hujita, Nonaka, & Oka (2006)	Propranolol	10		Broca's and Wernicke's aphasia	None specified	BNT, verbal fluency (FAS, vegetables)	Short-term beneficial effect on naming
Beversdorf et al. (2007)	Propranolol	4	CVA (ischemic)	Broca's Aphasia with anomia	None specified	BNT	Greater improvement in naming with propranolol than placebo
Tanaka et al. (2010)	Propranolol	11		Mild to moderate Broca's, Wernicke's, and amnestic aphasia	None specified	BNT, ANT, verbal fluency (category), auditory comp, BDAE Cookie Theft	Significant improvement for all subjects on BNT, ANT, verbal fluency and auditory comp tests; one month after discontinuation of propranolol scores returned to baseline
Tanaka et al. (2004)	Fluvoxamine vs. nilvadipine	10	CVA (ischemic, haemorrhagic)	Fluent aphasia; Wernicke's/jargon aphasia	None specified	WAB (Japanese version), BNT, ANT, word generation, BDAE, Token Test	Improvements in naming and mood, decreased perseveration with fluvoxamine (SSRI) for non-severe patients

(Continued)

TABLE 1
(Continued)

Author, year	Drug	N	Aetiology	Aphasia type & severity (pre-treatment)	Concurrent treatment	Linguistic outcome measures (pre- & post-treatment)	Results
Cohen, Chaaban, and Habert (2004)	Zolpidem	1	CVA	Severe Broca's aphasia	None specified	Non-standardised language exam	20 min after each administration, striking improvement of speech fluency, w/accurate and meaningful words, repetition of words, pseudo-words and short sentences
Laska, von Arbin, Kahan, Hellblom, and Murray (2005)	Moclobemide	90	CVA		None specified	Grunntest for afasi, Amsterdam-Nijmegen-everyday-language-test	No significance
Tsikunov and Belokoskova (2007)	Vasopressin	26	CVA (ischemic)	Acousto-agnostic and acousto-amnestic aphasia	None specified	Battery of speech-language subtests (e.g., naming, comprehension, repetition, spontaneous speech, verbal fluency, reading, etc)	Differential improvement in domains of speech/language depending on aphasia type
Jianu et al. (2010)	Cerebrolysin	156	CVA (ischemic)	Broca's aphasia	Standard therapy within 72 hours from stroke onset	Romanian WAB, NIHSS	Improvement in AQ, spontaneous speech, naming and repetition with adjuvant cerebrolysin treatment

Notes: **AQ**, Aphasia Quotient; **WAB**, Western Aphasia Battery; **PICA**, Porch Index of Communicative Ability; **BNT**, Boston Naming Test; **BDAE**, Boston Diagnostic Aphasia Examination; **ANT**, Action Naming Test; **PALPA**, Psycholinguistic Assessments of Language Processing in Aphasia; **RCPM**, Raven's Colored Progressive Matrices; **CAL**, Communicative Activity Log; **AAT**, Aachen Aphasia Test; **NIHSS**, National Institute of Health Stroke Scale; **RAN**, Rapid Automatised Naming; **CVA**, Cerebrovascular Accident; **TBI**, Traumatic Brain Injury; **TCMA**, Transcortical Motor Aphasia; **PPA**, Primary Progressive Aphasia; **SLT**, Speech-language Therapy; **CIAT**, Constraint-induced Aphasia Therapy; **MMSE**, Mini Mental State Exam; **SSRI**, Selective Serotonin Reuptake Inhibitor.

These outcome measures usually consist of scores on standardised tests, such as Boston Naming Test (Kaplan, 1983), Action Naming Test (Obler & Albert, 1979) and Verbal Fluency Test (Benton & Hamsher, 1976), which are clinically driven. The underlying assumption in these studies is that impairments in language fluency, comprehension, repetition, reading and writing will improve post-treatment based on aphasia classification and severity. These clinical distinctions might lack sufficient granularity to capture fine-grained language changes following treatment. We, thus, argue that in the absence of a clear psycholinguistic theoretical basis for task selection, the interpretability of pharmacotherapeutic effects on people with aphasia becomes difficult. We suggest using psycholinguistic models in conjunction with neurobiological approaches to aphasia recovery, to establish a clear rationale for the experimental design of aphasia pharmacotherapy studies, especially for the linguistic tasks chosen to measure treatment outcomes.

PSYCHOLINGUISTICS OF APHASIA PHARMACOTHERAPY: A NEW FRONTIER

How might one approach a pharmacotherapy study of aphasia from a psycholinguistic perspective? Rapp et al. (2013) considered a similar question in relation to aphasia treatment studies using neuroimaging techniques, which also face a comparable challenge of reconciling mixed, incongruent results. They identified crucial methodological prerequisites, which, if followed, would likely improve the experimental design of such studies, increasing interpretability of results. In what follows, then, we follow the rationale of Rapp et al. (2013), in proposing how psycholinguistic rigor can be applied in aphasia pharmacotherapy studies.

PSYCHOLINGUISTIC CONSIDERATIONS

A first step in identifying treatment-based language changes resulting from pharmacotherapy in people with aphasia would be the creation of a language profile of pre-treatment baseline performance, based on a given psycholinguistic theoretical framework. Such a profile would involve characterising pre-intervention impaired and spared functions, which could then be compared to post-intervention performance and allow for the identification of treatment-based effects. To isolate these treatment effects, the tasks selected should be designed to detect dissociations in the patterns of errors produced by study participants.

As Rapp et al. (2013) point out, when studying naming deficits, for example, a reasonable psycholinguistic framework could include the assumption that spoken word production engages multiple processes, distinguishing semantic, lexical, phonemic and motor production levels (e.g., Rapp & Goldrick, 2006). Thus, to identify whether or not a drug "improves" naming, the experimenters would first have to rule out impaired vision and hearing, semantic problems (e.g., by testing auditory comprehension) and motor problems (e.g., by testing repetition abilities). Then, they would need to be able to help determine which underlying psycholinguistic mechanism affects the naming errors produced—semantic and/or phonemic (e.g., by examining paraphasias and determining which cues are more helpful for increasing naming accuracy).

Rapp et al. (2013) caution that in order to reliably isolate treatment effects on language performance, pre- and post-intervention evaluations should also be accompanied by a comprehensive assessment of language-related cognitive domains, such as attention, working memory and executive functions. In principle, more precise characterisation of specific effects on language performance can be obtained if comparisons between experimental vs. control tasks are made (e.g., Caplan, 2009). However, from a neurochemical perspective, it is likely that pharmacological manipulation of a given neurotransmitter system will affect linguistic and, to some extent, other related cognitive processes, dependent on the functionality of its pathways. Thus, a psycholinguistic model which postulates interdependencies between linguistic operations and specific cognitive functions, such as attention, inhibition or set-shifting, will likely best predict patterns of deficits resulting from neural changes. Support for this idea comes from the growing literature describing the co-morbidity of different cognitive deficits and language impairment which can be observed among people with aphasia (e.g., Kurland, 2011; Martin & Reilly, 2012). Studies of language changes among healthy older adults also points in this direction, as executive functions, such as working memory and inhibitory control, have been associated with both preservation and decline of different language functions, such as sentence processing (e.g., Goral et al., 2011).

COMBINING PSYCHOLINGUISTICS AND NEUROBIOLOGY: THE CASE OF BETA-ADRENERGIC BLOCKING AGENTS

We offer here an example of the principal thesis being proposed in this paper: an integrative approach to aphasia pharmacotherapy could be used to investigate the efficacy of beta adrenergic drugs for the augmentation of language performance in people with aphasia. Preliminary evidence suggests that administration of a beta-blocking agent, such as propranolol, positively affects language performance in people with aphasia, improving, for example, their naming abilities (Beversdorf et al., 2007; Tanaka, Albert, Fujita, Nonaka, & Oka, 2007; Tanaka et al., 2010). Because such agents block the receptors for the physical effects involved in the natural "fight or flight" response (e.g., increased heart rate), inhibiting negative feelings of impending danger (e.g., anxiety), some researchers have speculated that beta blockers act to decrease autonomic nervous system (ANS) physiological responses (e.g., reduce heart rate) to improve language performance, in ways comparable to the amelioration of the phenomenon of "performance anxiety" in otherwise healthy individuals (Tanaka et al., 2010). Beta-adrenergic enhancement of naming has also been explained in terms of modulation of signal-to-noise ratio in the cortex (Hasselmo, Linster, Patil, Ma, & Cekic, 1997; Heilman, Nadeau, & Beversdorf, 2003), resulting in increased efficiency of information processing. Although these different theoretical accounts can potentially be teased apart by studies distinguishing peripheral and central autonomic components in persons with and without aphasia (Cahana-Amitay et al., 2011), they fail to make specific predictions as to the types of errors the pharmacological intervention might alleviate.

More explicit predictions about the consequences of ANS dysregulation can be made, for example, using Cahana-Amitay et al.'s (2011) framework of "linguistic anxiety" in aphasia, which postulates that altered ANS activity, as measured by stress-induced physiologic responses (e.g., changes in heart rate), can adversely affect language performance in aphasia, especially on tasks with heavy attention demands. In their view, people with aphasia who experience language use as a stressor (e.g., when speaking in front of strangers, when attempting to follow a conversation in noisy conditions) also demonstrate changes in physiologic stress reactivity, which might further impair their performance on the language task. This physiologic change is then assumed to lead to a resource allocation imbalance, whereby attention resources that would otherwise be allocated to task performance, are directed towards suppressing hyper-concerns about the challenges of the language task, continually reinforced by aroused physiologic stress responses. The most adverse effects on performance would be observed in situations where the processing of linguistic information in the presence of competing stimuli is required, as the suppression of worry would be competing for the same attention resources required for processing task-relevant information.

Given this theoretical framework, *the benefits of using beta-blocking agents to improve language performance among people with aphasia can be evaluated anew by examining changes in performance of language tasks involving inhibition of non-target competitors, as a result of the pharmacological intervention.* To identify pre- and post-treatment effects, it would be necessary first to assess the presence of physiologic stress reactivity, using physiologic biomarkers of ANS activity, such as heart rate variability, galvanic skin responses or blood pressure. Then, an evaluation of attention abilities would be required, to rule out a general attention dysfunction (e.g., sustained vigilance, working memory) that might interfere with language performance (for types of attention tasks that can be used to assess people with aphasia (see Connor & Fucetola, 2011). Finally, assessment of performance on language tasks with and without competing stimuli would have to be done, to determine whether they are differentially affected by treatment. The determination of what constitutes a "competing target" depends entirely on the research interests of the investigator. Competition can occur at any linguistic level—semantic, phonological, sentential and discursive—and affect many language functions, including language production, auditory comprehension and reading comprehension (e.g., Connor & Fucetola, 2011; Kurland, 2011).

Regardless of the source of linguistic competition, the research hypothesis would be that beta adrenergic manipulation would ameliorate performance of language tasks involving competing stimuli by targeting ANS biomarkers and freeing up attention resources taxed by the increased stress. Note that these treatment effects are expected to be more modest in people with a general attention dysfunction. In such people, attention problems are likely to be mediated by additional neurochemical mechanisms independent of those associated with increased stress, and so are less likely to improve in response to this particular pharmacological intervention. These people might respond better to pharmacotherapies directly targeting attention deficits (e.g., dopamine agonists). Speculations about such treatment effects cannot be made using scores on standardised language tasks, as those tests often lack the diagnostic sensitivity to differences in attention-processing demands and might therefore fail to reflect distinct-treatment effects.

ASKING THE RIGHT QUESTIONS

The extent to which psycholinguistics can inform aphasia pharmacotherapy studies is constrained by the degree to which language assessments that take psycholinguistic factors into account are utilised in aphasia therapy. Psycholinguistic models have been steadily working their way into aphasia treatment programs. Some treatments of naming impairment, for instance, have been based on a psycholinguistic model of semantic feature complexity that specifies exemplar typicality (e.g., Kiran & Johnson, 2008; Kiran & Thompson, 2003). Or, treatment of certain sentential deficits have been designed to reflect a language model differentiating sentence types by the level of syntactic complexity (e.g., Thompson, Den Ouden, Bonakdarpour, Garibaldi, & Parrish, 2010; Thompson & Shapiro, 2007; Thompson, Shapiro, Kiran, & Sobecks,

2003). These attempts bode well for the incorporation of psycholinguistic models into aphasia pharmacotherapy studies, promising to increase the resolution with which we can identify functional changes resulting from neurochemical manipulation of specific neurotransmitter systems.

This review paper has a specific, and limited, goal: to highlight psycholinguistic gaps in the current aphasia pharmacotherapy literature and to emphasise the importance of incorporating contemporary psycholinguistic knowledge into clinical research studies of aphasia pharmacotherapy. We do not wish to suggest that there should be a "one-size-fits-all" approach to the study of drug effects on language performance among people with aphasia. Clearly, single-case studies, small case series, controlled proof-of-principle experiments and controlled clinical trials have different goals and, therefore, distinct methodologies, each with its own strengths and shortcomings. Smaller-scale studies might, perhaps, lend themselves more easily to the exploration of fine-grained theoretically motivated dependent outcomes measuring language impairment.

If we take the examination of the effects of beta-adrenergic blocking agents on word retrieval as an example, one could imagine administration of an extensive language battery to up to twelve individuals, designed to measure baseline, mid-, and post-intervention performance, using accuracy scores and/or reaction times on tasks that vary in their processing demands. These tasks might include lexical decision tests with or without a competing distractor, cloze-completion tasks involving sentences that vary in syntactic complexity or noun and verb retrieval rates in discourse tasks with thematically linked content but differing discourse demands (e.g., examining nouns/verbs per minute in a stroke narrative vs. an expository opinion about treatment of stroke in the healthcare system). Results from such small-scale studies are likely to help determine which language measures most compellingly reflect treatment-induced changes in performance, which could then be incorporated into a larger-scale study. We recognise the many difficulties inherent in aphasia treatment studies, pharmacotherapeutic or others, but propose this new direction, nonetheless, as a challenge worth undertaking, as it may enable the detection of the beneficial effects of treatment not previously considered, that may have both theoretical and clinically meaningful consequences.

REFERENCES

Aarsland, D., Larsen, J. P., Reinvang, I., & Aasland, A. M. (1994). Effects of cholinergic blockade on language in healthy young women: Implications for the cholinergic hypothesis in dementia of the Alzheimer type. *Brain, 117*(6), 1377–1384. doi:10.1093/brain/117.6.1377

Albert, M. L. (1988). Neurobiological aspects of aphasia therapy. *Aphasiology, 2*(3–4), 215–218. doi:10.1080/02687038808248912

Albert, M. L. (2000). Toward a neurochemistry of naming and anomia. In Y. Grodzinsky, L. Shapiro, & D. Swinney (Eds.), *Language and the brain* (pp. 157–165). San Diego, CA: Academic Press.

Alexander, M. P. (2006). Impairments of procedures for implementing complex language are due to disruption of frontal attention processes. *Journal of the International Neuropsychological Society: JINS, 12*(2), 236–247. doi:10.1017/S1355617706060309

Angwin, A. J., Copland, D. A., Chenery, H. J., Murdoch, B. E., & Silburn, P. A. (2006). The influence of dopamine on semantic activation in Parkinson's disease. *Neuropsychology, 20*, 299–306.

Arciniegas, D. B., Frey, K. L., Anderson, C. A., Brousseau, K. M., & Harris, S. N. (2004). Amantadine for neurobehavioural deficits following delayed post-hypoxic encephalopathy. *Brain Injury, 18*(12), 1309–1318.

Ashtary, F., Janghorbani, M., Chitsaz, A., Reisi, M., & Bahrami, A. (2006). A randomized, double-blind trial of bromocriptine efficacy in nonfluent aphasia after stroke. *Neurology*, *66*(6), 914–916. doi:10.1212/01.wnl.0000203119.91762.0c

Barrett, A. M., & Eslinger, P. J. (2007). Amantadine for adynamic speech: Possible benefit for aphasia? *American Journal of Physical Medicine and Rehabilitation*, *86*(8), 605–612.

Benton, A. L., & Hamsher, K. (1976). *Multilingual aphasia examination*. Iowa: University of Iowa.

Berthier, M.L. (1999). *Transcortical aphasia*. Hove: Psychology Press.

Berthier, M. L. (2005). Poststroke aphasia: Epidemiology, pathophysiology and treatment. *Drugs & Aging*, *22*(2), 163–182.

Berthier, M. L., García-Casares, N., Walsh, S. F., Nabrozidis, A., de Mier, R. J. R., Green, C., . . . Pulvermüller, F. (2011). Recovery from post-stroke aphasia: Lessons from brain imaging and implications for rehabilitation and biological treatments. *Discovery Medicine*, *12*(65), 275–289.

Berthier, M. L., Green, C., Higueras, C., Fernández, I., Hinojosa, J., & Martín, M. C. (2006). A randomized, placebo-controlled study of donepezil in poststroke aphasia. *Neurology*, *67*(9), 1687–1689. doi:10.1212/01.wnl.0000242626.69666.e2

Berthier, M. L., Green, C., Lara, J. P., Higueras, C., Barbancho, M. A., Dávila, G., & Pulvermüller, F. (2009). Memantine and constraint-induced aphasia therapy in chronic poststroke aphasia. *Annals of Neurology*, *65*(5), 577–585. doi:10.1002/ana.21597

Berthier, M. L., Hinojosa, J., Martín, M. del C., & Fernández, I. (2003). Open-label study of donepezil in chronic poststroke aphasia. *Neurology*, *60*(7), 1218–1219. doi:10.1212/01.WNL.0000055871.82308.41

Berthier, M. L., Hinojosa, J., & Moreno-Torre, I. (2004). Beneficial effects of donepezil and modality-specific language therapy on chronic conduction aphasia. *Neurology*, *62*(Suppl 5), A462.

Berthier, M. L., & Pulvermüller, F. (2011). Neuroscience insights improve neurorehabilitation of poststroke aphasia. *Nature Reviews Neurology*, *7*(2), 86–97. doi:10.1038/nrneurol.2010.201

Beversdorf, D. Q., Narayanan, A., Hillier, A., & Hughes, J. D. (2007). Network model of decreased context utilization in autism spectrum disorder. *Journal of Autism and Developmental Disorders*, *37*(6), 1040–1048. doi:10.1007/s10803-006-0242-7

Bragoni, M., Altieri, M., Di Piero, V., Padovani, A., Mostardini, C., & Lenzi, G. L. (2000). Bromocriptine and speech therapy in non-fluent chronic aphasia after stroke. *Neurological Sciences: Official Journal of the Italian Neurological Society and of the Italian Society of Clinical Neurophysiology*, *21*(1), 19–22.

Breitenstein, C., Wailke, S., Bushuven, S., Kamping, S., Zwitserlood, P., Ringelstein, E. B., & Knecht, S. (2004). D-amphetamine boosts language learning independent of its cardiovascular and motor arousing effects. *Neuropsychopharmacology: Official Publication of the American College of Neuropsychopharmacology*, *29*(9), 1704–1714. doi:10.1038/sj.npp.1300464

Cahana-Amitay, D., Albert, M. L., Pyun, S.-B., Westwood, A., Jenkins, T., Wolford, S., & Finley, M. (2011). Language as a stressor in aphasia. *Aphasiology*, *25*(2), 593–614. doi:10.1080/02687038.2010.541469

Caplan, D. (2009). Experimental design and interpretation of functional neuroimaging studies of cognitive processes. *Human Brain Mapping*, *30*(1), 59–77. doi:10.1002/hbm.20489

Chen, Y., Li, Y.-S., Wang, Z.-Y., Xu, Q., Shi, G.-W., & Lin, Y. (2010). The efficacy of donepezil for post-stroke aphasia: A pilot case control study. *Zhonghua Nei Ke Za Zhi [Chinese Journal of Internal Medicine]*, *49*(2), 115–118.

Cherney, L. R., Erickson, R. K., & Small, S. L. (2010). Epidural cortical stimulation as adjunctive treatment for non-fluent aphasia: Preliminary findings. *Journal of Neurology, Neurosurgery, and Psychiatry*, *81*(9), 1014–1021. doi:10.1136/jnnp.2009.184036

Cohen, L., Chaaban, B., & Habert, M. O. (2004). Transient improvement of aphasia with zolpidem. *New England Journal of Medicine*, *350*(9), 949–950.

Connor, L. T., & Fucetola, R. P. (2011). Assessment of attention in people with aphasia: Challenges and recommendations. *Perspectives on Neurophysiology and Neurogenic Speech and Language Disorders*, *21*(2), 55–63. doi:10.1044/nnsld21.2.55

Corbett, F., Jefferies, E., & Lambon Ralph, M. A. (2008). The use of cueing to alleviate recurrent verbal perseverations: Evidence from transcortical sensory aphasia. *Aphasiology*, *22*(4), 363–382. doi:10.1080/02687030701415245

Crosson, B., Moore, A. B., Gopinath, K., White, K. D., Wierenga, C. E., Gaiefsky, M. E., . . . Gonzalez Rothi, L. J. (2005). Role of the right and left hemispheres in recovery of function during treatment of intention in aphasia. *Journal of Cognitive Neuroscience*, *17*(3), 392–406. doi:10.1162/0898929053279487

Darley, F. L., Keith, R. L., & Sasanuma, S. 1977. The effect of alerting and tranquilizing drugs on upon the performance of aphasic patients. *Clinical Aphasiology*, *7*, 91–96.

De Boissezon, X., Peran, P., De Boysson, C., & Démonet, J.-F. (2007). Pharmacotherapy of aphasia: Myth or reality? *Brain and Language, 102*(1), 114–125. doi:10.1016/j.bandl.2006.07.004

Floel, A., & Cohen, L. G. (2010). Recovery of function in humans: Cortical stimulation and pharmacological treatments after stroke. *Neurobiology of Disease, 37*(2), 243–251. doi:10.1016/j.nbd.2009.05.027

Gold, M., Van Dam, D., & Silliman, E. R. (2000). An open-label trial of bromocriptine in nonfluent aphasia: A qualitative analysis of word storage and retrieval. *Brain and Language, 74*(2), 141–156.

Goral, M., Clark-Cotton, M., Spiro, A., Obler, L. K., Verkuilen, J., & Albert, M. L. (2011). The contribution of set switching and working memory to sentence processing in older adults. *Experimental Aging Research, 37*(5), 516–538. doi:10.1080/0361073X.2011.619858

Gotts, S. J., Della Rocchetta, A. I., & Cipolotti, L. (2002). Mechanisms underlying perseveration in aphasia: Evidence from a single case study. *Neuropsychologia, 40*(12), 1930–1947. doi:10.1016/S0028-3932(02)00067-2

Güngör, L., Terzi, M., & Onar, M. K. (2011). Does long term use of piracetam improve speech disturbances due to ischemic cerebrovascular diseases? *Brain and Language, 117*(1), 23–27. doi:10.1016/j.bandl.2010.11.003

Gupta, S. R., & Mlcoch, A. G. (1992). Bromocriptine treatment of nonfluent aphasia. *Archives of Physical Medicine and Rehabilitation, 73*(4), 373–376.

Gupta, S. R., Mlcoch, A. G., Scolaro, C., & Moritz, T. (1995). Bromocriptine treatment of nonfluent aphasia. *Neurology, 45*, 2170–2173.

Hasselmo, M. E., Linster, C., Patil, M., Ma, D., & Cekic, M. (1997). Noradrenergic suppression of synaptic transmission may influence cortical signal-to-noise ratio. *Journal of Neurophysiology, 77*(6), 3326–3339.

Heilman, K. M., Nadeau, S. E., & Beversdorf, D. O. (2003). Creative innovation: Possible brain mechanisms. *Neurocase, 9*(5), 369–379. doi:10.1076/neur.9.5.369.16553

Heiss, W.-D., & Thiel, A. (2006). A proposed regional hierarchy in recovery of post-stroke aphasia. *Brain and Language, 98*(1), 118–123. doi:10.1016/j.bandl.2006.02.002

Hong, J. M., Shin, D. H., Lim, T. S., Lee, J. S., & Huh, K. (2012). Galantamine administration in chronic post-stroke aphasia. *Journal of Neurology, Neurosurgery, and Psychiatry, 83*, 675–680. doi: 10.1136/jnnp-2012-302268

Huber, W., Willmes, K., Poeck, K., Van Vleymen, B., & Deberdt, W. (1997). Piracetam as an adjuvant to language therapy for aphasia: A randomized double-blind placebo-controlled pilot study. *Archives of Physical Medicine and Rehabilitation, 78*(3), 245–250.

Jianu, D. C., Muresanu, D. F., Bajenaru, O., Popescu, B. O., Deme, S. M., Moessler, H., . . . Ursoniu, S. (2010). Cerebrolysin adjuvant treatment in Broca's aphasics following first acute ischemic stroke of the left middle cerebral artery. *Journal of Medicine and Life, 3*(3), 297–307.

Johnson, N. A., Rademaker, A., Weintraub, S., Gitelman, D., Wienecke, C., & Mesulam, M. (2010). Pilot trial of memantine in primary progressive aphasia. *Alzheimer Disease and Associated Disorders, 24*(3), 308.

Kaplan, E. (1983). *Boston naming test.* Philadelphia, PA: Lea & Febiger.

Kertesz, A., Morlog, D., Light, M., Blair, M., Davidson, W., Jesso, S., & Brashear, R. 2008. Galantamine in frontotemporal dementia and primary progressive aphasia. *Dementia and Geriatric Cognitive Disorders, 25*, 178–185.

Kertesz, A., Sheppard, A., & MacKenzie, R. (1982). Localization in transcortical sensory aphasia. *Archives of Neurology, 39*(8), 475–478.

Kessler, J., Thiel, A., Karbe, H., & Heiss, W. D. (2000). Piracetam improves activated blood flow and facilitates rehabilitation of poststroke aphasic patients. *Stroke; A Journal of Cerebral Circulation, 31*(9), 2112–2116.

Kiran, S., & Johnson, L. (2008). Semantic complexity in treatment of naming deficits in aphasia: Evidence from well-defined categories. *American Journal of Speech-Language Pathology, 17*(4), 389–400. doi:10.1044/1058–0360(2008/06–0085

Kiran, S., & Thompson, C. K. (2003). The role of semantic complexity in treatment of naming deficits: Training semantic categories in fluent aphasia by controlling exemplar typicality. *Journal of Speech, Language, and Hearing Research, 46*(4), 773–787. doi:10.1044/1092-4388(2003/061

Klein, R. B., & Albert, M. L. (2004). Can drug therapies improve language functions of individuals with aphasia? A review of the evidence. *Seminars in Speech and Language, 25*(2), 193–204. doi:10.1055/s-2004-825655

Knecht, S., Breitenstein, C., Bushuven, S., Wailke, S., Kamping, S., Flöel, A., . . . Ringelstein, E. B. (2004). Levodopa: Faster and better word learning in normal humans. *Annals of Neurology, 56*(1), 20–26. doi:10.1002/ana.20125

Kurland, J. (2011). The role that attention plays in language processing. *Perspectives on Neurophysiology and Neurogenic Speech and Language Disorders*, *21*(2), 47–54.

Laska, A. C., von Arbin, M., Kahan, T., Hellblom, A., & Murray, V. (2005). Long-term antidepressant treatment with moclobemide for aphasia in acute stroke patients: A randomised, double-blind, placebo-controlled study. *Cerebrovascular Diseases*, *19*(2), 125–132.

Lazar, R. M., & Antoniello, D. (2008). Variability in recovery from aphasia. *Current Neurology and Neuroscience Reports*, *8*(6), 497–502.

Lee, A. W., & Hillis, A. E. (2008). The pharmacological treatment of aphasia. In B. Stemmer & H. A. Whitaker (Eds.), *Handbook of the neuroscience of language* (pp. 407–415). London: Academic Press.

Leeman, B., Laganaro, M., Chetelat-Mabillard, D., & Schnider, A. (2011). Crossover trial of subacute computerized aphasia therapy for anomia with the addition of either levodopa or placebo. *Neurorehabilitation and Neural Repair*, *25*(1), 43–47.

Luriiâ, A. R. (1970). *Traumatic aphasia: Its syndromes, psychology and treatment*. The Hague: Mouton.

MacLennan, D. L., Nicholas, L. E., Morley, G. K., & Brookshire, R. H. (1991). The effects of bromocriptine on speech and language function in a man with transcortical aphasia. *Clinical Aphasiology*, *21*, 145–155.

Martin, N., & Reilly, J. J. (2012). Introduction to special issue. Short-term memory/working memory impairments in aphasia: Data, models and their application to aphasia rehabilitation. *Aphasiology*, *26*(3/4), 253–257.

McNamara, P., & Albert, M. L. (2004). Neuropharmacology of verbal perseveration. *Seminars in Speech and Language*, *25*(4), 309–321. doi:10.1055/s-2004-837244

McNeil, M. R., Doyle, P. J., Spencer, K. A., Goda, A. J., Flores, D., & Small, S. L. (1997). A double-blind, placebo-controlled study of pharmacological and behavioural treatment of lexical-semantic deficits in aphasia. *Aphasiology*, *11*(4–5), 385–400.

McNeil, M. R., Small, S. L., Masterson, R. J., & Fossett, T. R. D. (1995). Behavioral and pharmacological treatment of lexical-semantic deficits in a single patient with primary progressive aphasia. *American Journal of Speech-Language Pathology*, *4*(4), 76–87.

Mimura, M., Albert, M. L., & McNamara, P. (1995). Toward a pharmacotherapy for aphasia. In H. Kirshner (Ed.), *Handbook of neurological speech and language disorders* (pp. 465–482). New York, NY: Marcel Dekker.

Nadeau, S. E., & Wu, S. S. (2006). CIMT as a behavioral engine in research on physiological adjuvants to neurorehabilitation: The challenge of merging animal and human research. *NeuroRehabilitation*, *21*(2), 107–130.

Obler, L. K., & Albert, M. L. (1979). *The action naming test* (experimental edition). Boston, MA: VA Medical Center.

Orgogozo, J. M. (1999). Piracetam in the treatment of acute stroke. *Pharmacopsychiatry*, *32*(Suppl. 1), 25–32.

Ozeren, A., Sarica, Y., Mavi, H., & Demirkiran, M. (1995). Bromocriptine is ineffective in the treatment of chronic nonfluent aphasia. *Acta Neurologica Belgica*, *95*(4), 235–238.

Pashek, G. V., & Bachman, D. L. (2003). Cognitive, linguistic, and motor speech effects of donepezil hydrochloride in a patient with stroke-related aphasia and apraxia of speech. *Brain and Language*, *87*, 179–180.

Pulvermüller, F., Neininger, B., Elbert, T., Mohr, B., Rockstroh, B., Koebbel, P., & Taub, E. (2001). Constraint-induced therapy of chronic aphasia after stroke. *Stroke; A Journal of Cerebral Circulation*, *32*(7), 1621–1626.

Rapp, B., Caplan, D., Edwards, S., Visch-Brink, E., & Thompson, C. K. (2013). Neuroimaging in aphasia treatment research: Issues of experimental design for relating cognitive to neural changes. *NeuroImage*, *73*, 200–207. doi:10.1016/j.neuroimage.2012.09.007

Rapp, B., & Goldrick, M. (2006). Speaking words: Contributions of cognitive neuropsychological research. *Cognitive Neuropsychology*, *23*(1), 39–73. doi:10.1080/02643290542000049

Raymer, A. M. (2003). Treatment of adynamia in aphasia. *Frontiers in Bioscience: A Journal and Virtual Library*, *8*, s845–s851.

Raymer, A. M., Bandy, D., Adair, J. C., Schwartz, R. L., Williamson, D. J., Gonzalez Rothi, L. J., & Heilman, K. M. (2001). Effects of bromocriptine in a patient with crossed nonfluent aphasia: A case report. *Archives of Physical Medicine and Rehabilitation*, *82*(1), 139–144. doi:10.1053/apmr.2001.18056

Reed, D. A., Johnson, N. A., Thompson, C., Weintraub, S., & Mesulam, M. M. (2004). A clinical trial of bromocriptine for treatment of primary progressive aphasia. *Annals of Neurology*, *56*(5), 750. doi: 10.1002/ana.20301

Sabe, L., Leiguarda, R., & Starkstein, S. E. (1992). An open-label trial of bromocriptine in nonfluent aphasia. *Neurology, 42*, 1637–1638.

Sabe, L., Salvarezza, F., García Cuerva, A., Leiguarda, R., & Starkstein, S. (1995). A randomized, double-blind, placebo-controlled study of bromocriptine in nonfluent aphasia. *Neurology, 45*(12), 2272–2274.

Sarter, M., Hasselmo, M. E., Bruno, J. P., & Givens, B. (2005). Unraveling the attentional functions of cortical cholinergic inputs: Interactions between signal-driven and cognitive modulation of signal detection. *Brain Research Brain Research Reviews, 48*(1), 98–111. doi:10.1016/j.brainresrev.2004.08.006

Seniów, J., Litwin, M., Litwin, T., Leśniak, M., & Członkowska, A. (2009). New approach to the rehabilitation of post-stroke focal cognitive syndrome: Effect of levodopa combined with speech and language therapy on functional recovery from aphasia. *Journal of the Neurological Sciences, 283*(1–2), 214–218. doi:10.1016/j.jns.2009.02.336

Shisler, R. J., Baylis, G. C., & Frank, E. M. (2000). Pharmacological approaches to the treatment and prevention of aphasia. *Aphasiology, 14*(12), 1163–1186. doi:10.1080/02687030050205705

Small, S. L. (1994). Pharmacotherapy of aphasia. A critical review. *Stroke, 25*(6), 1282–1289. doi:10.1161/01.STR.25.6.1282

Small, S. L. (2000). The future of aphasia treatment. *Brain and Language, 71*(1), 227–232. doi:10.1006/brln.1999.2256S

Small, S. L., & Llano, D. A. (2009). Biological approaches to aphasia treatment. *Current Neurology and Neuroscience Reports, 9*(6), 443–450. doi:10.1007/s11910-009-0066-x

Sommer, I. E. C., Oranje, B., Ramsey, N. F., Klerk, F. A., Mandl, R. C. W., Westenberg, H. G. M., & Kahn, R. S. (2006). The influence of amphetamine on language activation: An fMRI study. *Psychopharmacology, 183*(4), 387–393. doi:10.1007/s00213-005-0176-3

Tanaka, Y., & Albert, M. L. (2001). *Cholinergic therapy for fluent aphasia*. Presented at the Annual Meeting of American Neurological Association, Chicago, IL.

Tanaka, Y., Albert, M. L., Aketa, S., Hujita, K., Noda, E., Takashima, M., . . . Tanaka, M. (2004). Serotonergic therapy for fluent aphasia. *Neurology, 62*(7, Suppl. S5), A166.

Tanaka, Y., Albert, M. L., Fujita, K., Nonaka, C., & Oka, T. (2007). Beta blocker improves language output in aphasia. *Neurological Medicine (Japan), 67*, 277–281.

Tanaka, Y., Albert, M. L., Hujita, F., Nonaka, C., & Oka, T. (2006). *Beta-blocker improves language output in aphasia*. Presented at the Annual Meeting of the American Neurological Association, Chicago, IL.

Tanaka, Y., Cahana-Amitay, D., Albert, M., Fujita, K., Nonaka, C., & Miyazaki, M. (2010). Treatment of anxiety in aphasia. *Procedia Social and Behavioral Sciences, 6*, 252–253. doi:10.1016/j.sbspro.2010.08.061

Tanaka, Y., Miyazaki, M., & Albert, M. L. (1997). Effects of increased cholinergic activity on naming in aphasia. *The Lancet, 350*(9071), 116–117. doi:10.1016/S0140-6736(05)61820-X

Thompson, C. K., Den Ouden, D.-B., Bonakdarpour, B., Garibaldi, K., & Parrish, T. B. (2010). Neural plasticity and treatment-induced recovery of sentence processing in agrammatism. *Neuropsychologia, 48*(11), 3211–3227. doi:10.1016/j.neuropsychologia.2010.06.036

Thompson, C. K., & Shapiro, L. P. (2007). Complexity in treatment of syntactic deficits. *American Journal of Speech-Language Pathology, 16*(1), 30–42. doi:10.1044/1058-0360(2007/005

Thompson, C. K., Shapiro, L. P., Kiran, S., & Sobecks, J. (2003). The role of syntactic complexity in treatment of sentence deficits in agrammatic aphasia: The complexity account of treatment efficacy (CATE). *Journal of Speech, Language, and Hearing Research, 46*(3), 591–607.

Tsikunov, S. G., & Belokoskova, S. G. (2007). Psychophysiological analysis of the influence of vasopressin on speech in patients with post-stroke aphasia. *The Spanish Journal of Psychology, 10*(1), 178–188.

Walker-Batson, D., Curtis, S., Natarajan, R., Ford, J., Dronkers, N., Salmeron, E., . . . Unwin, D. H. (2001). A double-blind, placebo-controlled study of the use of amphetamine in the treatment of aphasia. *Stroke, 32*(9), 2093–2098. doi:10.1161/hs0901.095720

Walker-Batson, D., Unwin, H., Curtis, S., Allen, E., Wood, M., Smith, P., . . . Greenlee, R. G. (1992). Use of amphetamine in the treatment of aphasia. *Restorative Neurology and Neuroscience, 4*(1), 47–50. doi:10.3233/RNN-1992-4106

Whiting, E., Chenery, H. J., Chalk, J., & Copland, D. A. (2007). Dexamphetamine boosts naming treatment effects in chronic aphasia. *Journal of the International Neuropsychological Society: JINS, 13*(6), 972–979. doi:10.1017/S1355617707071317

Dopaminergic therapy in aphasia

Sumanjit K. Gill[1] and Alexander P. Leff[2,3]

[1] Department of Medicine, Watford General Hospital, Watford, UK
[2] Institute of Cognitive Neuroscience, University College London, London, UK
[3] Department of Brain Repair and Rehabilitation, Institute of Neurology, University College London, London, UK

Background: The dopaminergic system is involved in a wide range of cognitive functions including motor control, reward, memory, attention, problem-solving and learning. This has stimulated interest in investigating the potential of dopaminergic drugs as cognitive enhancers in aphasic patients.

Aim: To discuss the evidence for the use of dopaminergic agents in patients with aphasia. Levodopa (L-dopa) and the dopamine agonist bromocriptine are the two drugs that have been trialled to date. We discuss, in some detail, the 15 studies that have been published on this topic from the first case report in 1988 to the present (2012), and assess the evidence from each.

Main contribution: In addition to summarising the effectiveness of the drugs that have been tried, we examine the possible cognitive mechanisms by which dopaminergic drugs may act on language function and aphasia recovery. Given the wide range of dopaminergic drugs, it is surprising that such a narrow range has been trialled in aphasic patients. Important lessons are to be learned from published studies and we discuss optimal trial designs to help guide future work.

Conclusions: The evidence for the efficacy of dopaminergic agents in aphasia therapy is mixed. Further trials with better tolerated agents are required. Optimal trial designs with appropriate control groups or blocks should be used. The mechanism of action is unclear, but at the cognitive level the evidence points towards either (re)learning of word-forms or their improved retrieval.

Levodopa (L-dopa) and the dopamine agonist bromocriptine are the two main drugs that have been trialled to date in patients with acquired aphasia. These studies were prompted by the observation that some Parkinsonian patients noted improved speech function following L-dopa therapy (Quaglieri & Celesia, 1977). Subsequent studies in patients with Parkinson's disease have shown that dopamine therapy can modulate the motoric aspects of speech: articulation and phonation, see (Goberman & Coelho, 2002) for a review of this literature; as well as the more linguistic aspects, verbal fluency (Gotham, Brown, & Marsden, 1988) and even sentence comprehension (Grossman et al., 2001). In post-stroke aphasia, the first reported use of dopaminergic therapy was bromocriptine used in a 62-year-old patient with a severe transcortical motor aphasia following a left frontal intracerebral haemorrhage 3.5 years prior to therapy. The bromocriptine caused a small improvement in his confrontation naming (5–10%) with a more marked improvement of the fluency of his spontaneous speech, and pauses between utterances were reduced by 24% (Albert, Bachman, Morgan, & Helm-Estabrooks, 1988). Single-case studies are often difficult to interpret, but if more than one period of "off–drug" is included, this helps. In this case, the patient's language function returned to baseline after cessation of therapy.

Before examining the rest of the literature, we will provide a quick pharmacological and anatomical resume of the dopaminergic system in humans. Dopamine is a monoamine neurotransmitter whose function was first characterised in 1958 (Benes, 2001). It is synthesised from L-3,4-dihydroxyphenylalanine (L-dopa), 95% of which is turned into dopamine by the action of the enzyme dopa-decarboxylase. The remaining 5% is then converted to noradrenaline and acts on adrenergic receptors. Dopamine acts on five subtypes of the dopamine receptor; however, these receptors fall into two main groups based on morphological grounds: D2-like (D2–D4: primarily located in the striatal neurons) and D1-like (D1 and D5: primarily located in the cortical neurons) (Civelli, Bunzow, & Grandy, 1993). Endogenous dopamine is mainly produced by two paired, midbrain nuclei which are situated close to each other: the ventral tegmental area (VTA) and substantia nigra (SN). Both project to different parts of the striatum and indirectly affect the cortical neurons via cortico-basal ganglia circuits, although the VTA also projects directly to prefrontal cortex (Figure 1(a)). A widespread subpopulation of cortical neurons also have dopamine receptors, so exogenous dopamine, particularly the receptor agonists and antagonists, have two main routes to affect the behaviour; either directly, or through existing cortico-basal ganglia circuits. Dopamine has been implicated in modulating a whole range of cognitive functions: motor control, reward, memory, attention, problem-solving and learning (Alexander, DeLong, & Strick, 1986) and could potentially affect language recovery through any or all of these.

The relative affinity of each dopamine agonist for each receptor subtype provides both its therapeutic effect and unwanted side effects. For example, the motor improvement seen in Parkinson's patients is attributed to the stimulation of D_2 receptors in the caudate and putamen, as are the unwanted end of dose deterioration and dyskinesias (Kvernmo, Hartter, & Burger, 2006). Perhaps surprisingly, the only dopamine agonist trialled in aphasic patients to date is bromocriptine. Bromocriptine is primarily a D2 receptor agonist with some D1 receptor antagonist properties (Kvernmo et al., 2006).

TRIAL EVIDENCE

Interest in dopaminergic effects on language recovery stemmed from the single-case study by Albert et al. (1988) and discussed above. The better trials have tended to be those with larger numbers and included a placebo-controlled arm. Without a placebo arm, patients always know when they are on the active drug so placebo effects can muddy the picture. Even with a placebo, not all trials blind the patient to this information (open-label trials). Some form of control arm or block is always preferable because most patients are on an upward recovery curve. Even though "spontaneous" recovery slows three months post infarct (Lazar et al., 2010; Lomas & Kertesz,

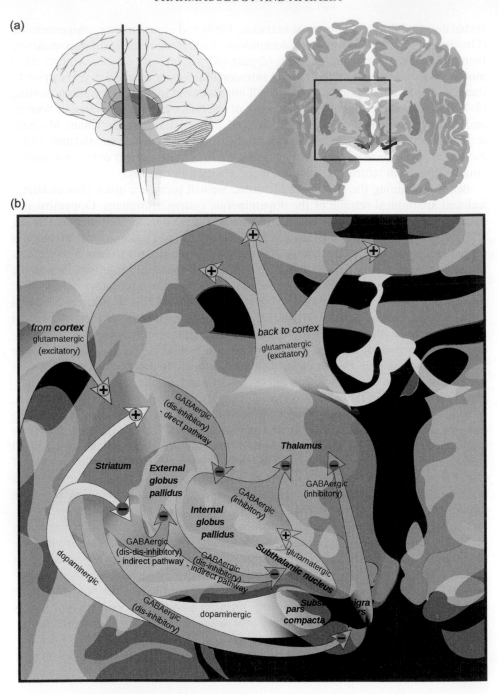

Figure 1. (a) The two main dopaminergic nuclei are close to each other in the midbrain with the substantia nigra projecting to the striatum and the ventral tegmental area projecting to both the nucleus accumbens (part of the ventral striatum) and the frontal cortex. (b) The nigrostriatal pathway affects cortical function indirectly through a series of cortico-basal ganglia circuits. The substantia nigra (pars compacta) projects to the striatum (caudate and putamen in blue). The main output of the striatum is to the globus pallidus (green) and thence to the thalamus (pink) and cortex (green arrows). The cortex feeds back to the striatum (green arrows) to close the loop on the cortico-basal ganglia circuits. There are also dopaminergic receptors on many cortical neurons (not shown). http://en.wikipedia.org/wiki/File:Basal_ganglia_circuits.svg. Mikael Häggström, based on images by Andrew Gillies.

1978), therapy-driven improvements in aphasia are reported in the chronic phase, even decades after the stroke occurred (Moss & Nicholas, 2006; Price, Seghier, & Leff, 2010). All but three of the trials reported here were performed in the chronic phase (defined as >6 months post-stroke); there is good evidence that treatments aimed at improving language outcomes are effective in this latter time period (Allen, Mehta, McClure, & Teasell, 2012). The 15 studies in aphasic patients (the vast majority with stroke) covered by this review are summarised in Table 1. Relevant studies were found by searching PubMED and Google Scholar using the following terms: aphasia, anomia, bromocriptine, dopaminergic, drug therapy, L-dopa, levodopa and rehabilitation. Two single cases, both reported in books, were highlighted by one of the referees. We will discuss them in chronological order.

Bromocriptine has been the drug of choice in 13 of the 15 studies. In Parkinson's disease, a dose range of 10–30 mg is usual, although bromocriptine has somewhat fallen out of favour with movement disorder specialists who prefer the newer dopamine agonists such as pramipexole and ropinirole. While bromocriptine is considered to be an effective treatment for Parkinson's disease, movement disorder specialists generally avoid all ergot-derived dopamine agonists because of the risks of lung fibrosis and heart valvulopathies (Dr Prasad Korlipara, Personal communication, 8 March 2013; Andersohn & Garbe, 2009). In order to minimise the occurrence of side effects, most studies employed an escalating dose regime up to 10 mg/day. Most titrated to between 10–30 mg but one group preferred to escalate to 60 mg. In the latter of their two studies, four of the seven patients taking part (57%) suffered side effects of nausea, dystonic movements or a lack of energy in the bromocriptine block (Sabe, Salvarezza, Garcia Cuerva, Leiguarda, & Starkstein, 1995). Another study with 11 patients titrated to 30 mg/day had a 63% incidence of side effects (Bragoni et al., 2000).

In 1991, MacLennan reported a case similar to the Albert one, although they used an AB and not an ABA design, which makes it difficult to interpret. Like the Albert case, there was no statistical treatment of the behavioural data, but there were two methodological improvements: a placebo was used with the subject blinded to the order of placebo/bromocriptine therapy, and a simple motor reaction time test was used to gauge any motoric effects of bromocriptine. There was no convincing effect of bromocriptine on motoric reaction time, naming or word fluency. The patient produced about 50% more words on a test of spoken picture description, with this effect continuing into the drug withdrawal phase. It is difficult to interpret this as the drug effect could be confounded by practice effects. The authors themselves concluded that the study was negative although, interestingly, the patient did not agree (MacLennan, Morley, & Brookshire, 1991).

In 1992, Gupta and Mlcoch (1992) went one better than the papers by Albert and MacLennan and reported a positive effect of bromocriptine in two aphasic patients with nonfluent aphasia in the chronic phase. Using an AB design (but no placebo block), both were started on bromocriptine and escalated from 10 mg to 30 mg/day. The main outcome measure was mean length of utterance, derived from an analysis of spoken picture description. The first patient showed some improvement in fluency at 10 mg and marked improvement at 30 mg, but it is difficult to rule out a simple time-effect (they perhaps should have tested him with an ABA design like Albert). The second patient's results were more interesting; he improved at 10 mg, got worse at 30 mg and improved again at 10 mg suggesting that, if the effect was due to the

TABLE 1

Summary of the 15 studies covered by this review

Title, 1st author, year	Trial type	Drug and dose	No. Pts	Aphasia type and chronicity	Main outcomes, comments
Pharmacotherapy for aphasia. Albert (1988).	Single case, no placebo, ABA design.	Bromocriptine, 15 then 30 mg	1	Transcortical motor aphasia. 3.5 years post-stroke.	Paired with therapy. Reduced hesitancy, decreased paraphrasias and increased naming ability. Return to baseline after cessation of therapy.
The effects of bromocriptine on speech and language function in a man with transcortical motor aphasia. MacLennan, 1990.	Single case, placebo-controlled, single blinded. AB design.	Bromocriptine 2.5 mg increased to 15 mg	1	Transcortical motor aphasia. 4 years post-stroke.	An increase in no. words and correct information units, but no statistical analysis made. Changes could be due to practice or carry-over effects.
Bromocriptine treatment of non-fluent aphasia. Gupta (1992).	Two cases, no placebo, AB design.	Bromocriptine, escalated dose: 10 mg, 30 mg	2	1 = Broca's aphasia; 1 = transcortical motor aphasia. 18 months and 10 years post-stroke.	Drug alone, not paired with therapy. Fluency of speech improved in both. In the second case worse on 30 mg and improved when dose deescalated to 10 mg.
An open label trial of bromocriptine in non-fluent aphasia. Sabe (1992).	No placebo, ABA ramp-up, ramp-down design.	Bromocriptine, up to 60 mg/day	7	4 = transcortical motor aphasia; 2 = Broca's aphasia; 1 = global aphasia. >1 year post-stroke.	Paired with therapy. An improvement seen in those who were moderately affected (4:3) with increased word finding and verbal fluency increasing on drug compared with baseline and then decreasing as the drug was withdrawn.
A randomised, double blind, placebo controlled study of bromocriptine in non-fluent aphasia. Sabe (1995).	Randomised*, double-blind, placebo-controlled, crossover design.	Bromocriptine, up to 60 mg/day	7	2 = Broca's aphasia; 3 = transcortical motor aphasia; 2 = anomic aphasia. >1 year post-stroke.	No benefit measured over placebo in hesitancy, verbal naming, verbal fluency, content words or content units. High rate of side effects in therapy block (57%) compared with control block (0%).

(Continued)

TABLE 1
(Continued)

Title, 1st author, year	Trial type	Drug and dose	No. Pts	Aphasia type and chronicity	Main outcomes, comments
Bromocriptine treatment of non-fluent aphasia. Gupta (1995).	Double-blind, placebo-controlled, crossover design.	Bromocriptine, up to 15 mg/day	20	7 = transcortical motor aphasia; 4 = Broca's aphasia; 9 = "mixed anterior aphasia". >1 year post-stroke.	Drug alone, not paired with therapy (therapy was not allowed during the trial). No improvement in speech fluency, language content, overall aphasia severity or non-verbal cognitive problems.
Bromocriptine is ineffective in the treatment of chronic non-fluent aphasia. Ozeren (1995).	No placebo, AB design.	Bromocriptine, 10–25 mg/day	4	2 = Broca's aphasia; 1 = transcortical motor aphasia; 1 = global. 24 to 35 months post-stroke.	No significant improvements on "aphasia tests" (a speech sample rated on an ordinal scale of three points). Outcome measure almost certainly not sensitive to change.
Transcortical motor aphasia. Berthier (1999).	Single case, no placebo, AB design.	Bromocriptine, titrated to 20 mg/day	1	Transcortical motor aphasia. Bilateral striatocapsular strokes (12 and 5 months prior to study) with Parkinsonian features.	Patient improved markedly on spoken picture description and aphasia quotient of the WAB. Mixture of improvements in Parkinsonian (motoric) and word finding aspects of speech.
An open label trial of bromocriptine in non-fluent aphasia: a qualitative analysis of word storage and retrieval. Gold (2000).	No placebo, ABBA design.	Bromocriptine, 15 mg/day	4	2 = Broca's aphasia; 2 = transcortical motor aphasia. 7 to 78 months post-stroke.	Drug alone, not paired with SALT. A significant improvement in word retrieval for all four on bromocriptine therapy with three experiencing decreases after withdrawal.

(Continued)

TABLE 1
(Continued)

Title, 1st author, year	Trial type	Drug and dose	No. Pts	Aphasia type and chronicity	Main outcomes, comments
Bromocriptine and speech therapy in nonfluent chronic aphasia after stroke. Bragoni (2000).	Double-blind placebo-controlled, but not randomised (placebo 1st block; bromocriptine 2nd block).	Bromocriptine, 30 mg/day	11(5#)	9 = Broca's aphasia; 2 = global aphasia. 6 to 96 months post-stroke.	Improved dictation, reading-comprehension, repetition and verbal latency but only 5/11 completed the study. Supposedly double-blind but high level of side effects. Placebo-controlled but not block-randomised.
Effects of bromocriptine in a patient with crossed non-fluent aphasia: a case report. Raymer (2001).	Single case, no placebo, ABABA design.	Bromocriptine, escalating dose up to 20 mg/day	1	Transcortical motor aphasia. NB: right frontal stroke involving IFG. 2 months post-stroke.	Improved verbal fluency sustained during withdrawal phases —this could have been due to spontaneous recovery.
A clinical trial of bromocriptine for treatment of primary progressive aphasia. Reed (2004).	Randomised, double-blinded, placebo-controlled, crossover.	Bromocriptine, 22.5 mg per day	6	Primary progressive aphasia (mean age 66.8 years).	Increased mean length of utterance but no effect on fluency or naming. Suggests a slowing of decline of the motoric aspects of speech.
A randomised double blind trial of bromocriptine efficacy in non-fluent aphasia after stroke. Ashtary (2006).	Randomised, double-blind, placebo-controlled.	Bromocriptine, up to 10 mg/day	38	Non-fluent aphasic patients, Persian speakers, in the "acute" phase.	Patients in both groups (placebo and bromocriptine) improved on all measures. No significant differences between the groups.
New approach to the rehabilitation of post-stroke focal cognitive syndrome: effect of levodopa combined with speech and language therapy on functional recovery from aphasia. Seniow (2009).	Randomised, double-blind, placebo-controlled.	L-dopa, 100 mg/day. Used in a phasic manner and paired with SALT	39	Any aphasia subtype. Acute phase (~5 weeks post-stroke). In-patients.	Increased naming and repetition on L-dopa compared with placebo. First study to attempt a sub-group analysis on lesion site (patients with "anterior" lesions responded better to L-dopa).

(Continued)

TABLE 1
(Continued)

Title, 1st author, year	Trial type	Drug and dose	No. Pts	Aphasia type and chronicity	Main outcomes, comments
Crossover trial of subacute computerised aphasia therapy for anomia with the addition of either levodopa or placebo. Leeman, Laganaro, Chetelat-Mabillard, and Schnider (2011).	Randomised, double-blind, placebo-controlled, crossover.	L-dopa, 100 mg/day. Used in a phasic manner and paired with computerised therapy and SALT.	12	2 = Broca's; 2 = Wernicke's; 6 = anomic; 1 = conduction. Acute (~7.5 weeks) Post-stroke (9) or traumatic brain injury (3). In-patients.	Significant improvements on the treated items from the computerised therapy battery but no interaction with drug/placebo block.

*Although reported as randomised (block randomised), all 7 patients were randomised to drug first then placebo. See text for further comment.
#High drop-out rate (54%). Only 5 completed the study.

drug, the patient may have been affected by the inverted "U" shape curve described in drug-based cognitive enhancement (Husain & Mehta, 2011).

In the same year, Sabe , Leiguarda, and Starkstein (1992) reported an open-label trial in seven patients with mixed aphasia type and severity according to the Western Aphasia Battery (WAB) (Kertesz, 1982): four moderate, three severe. The trial was effectively an ABA design with language tests at eight consecutive time points (every 2 weeks) as the dose of bromocriptine was ramped up and then down (0, 15, 30, 45, 60, 30, 15, 0 mg). This sort of design is reasonable as any time effects or familiarity with the language tests should be dissociable from drug effects when the dose ramps down. In theory this type of study can be blinded (patients blinded to the dose), but it looks like this was not the case. Conventional Speech and Language Therapy (SALT) was administered as well. One has to interpret the results with caution as the numbers were small, so inferences to the reference population (all aphasic patients of this type) must necessarily be limited, but they did show convincing dose effects in the moderate group's lexical index scores (a measure of correct word production in a composite picture description task), verbal fluency and pauses >3 seconds (a measure of speech fluency). So some patients improved on a mixture of tests that could reflect improved word retrieval, spoken fluency (motor) or non-specific effects such as attention. The study was not placebo-controlled or blinded, so the authors followed it up with a better designed study that was published three years later (Sabe et al., 1995). This also had the same number of patients in the chronic phase but who were less variable in terms of severity than the original study, all being in the moderate range on the WAB. A similar escalation of bromocriptine as in the 1992 study (6 weeks on drug) was used, but this time with no ramp-down, just a 3-week washout and then moving into the next block (6 weeks on placebo). Language outcome measures were taken weekly. In theory, this was a better designed study than the 1992 one; however, inexplicably, all patients were allocated to the "bromocriptine first" group. The chances of this happening are 0.5^7 or 1/128, so either they were very unlucky or something went wrong with their randomisation procedure. In small studies, it is a good idea to use block randomisation to avoid this (Lachin, Matts, & Wei, 1988). While they did employ a crossover design, the failure of random allocation of block order meant that time effects were conflated with treatment effects although the study was negative, with no significant drug (or time) effects found for any of the language outcome measures.

In the same issue of *Neurology*, Gupta et al. (1995) reported the findings of their larger study with 20 patients at least 1 year post-stroke, median = 3 years (Gupta, Mlcoch, Scolaro, & Moritz, 1995). This was a follow-on study from their 1992 paper with two patients. They escalated the bromocriptine dose by 5 mg a week to 15 mg which was given for 6 weeks followed by a 6-week washout. A crossover design was employed with patients randomised to placebo first ($n = 9$) or bromocriptine first ($n = 11$). SALT was prohibited during the trial so this was the first group study to investigate dopaminergic effects independent of concomitant SALT. The trial was well conducted; there were five evaluation periods, three at times when subjects were drug/placebo-free so test-learning effects could be evaluated (and discounted). Outcomes included language assessments (WAB, Boston naming tests and a transcription of conversational speech) and cognitive assessments (Wechsler Memory Scale, Raven's Progressive Matrices and the Rey–Osterrieth Figure). There were no significant effects (drug vs. placebo) on any of these outcome measures. The year 1995 was a busy one and saw the publication of a third study that was also negative, although only four patients took part (Ozeren, Sarica, Mavi, & Demirkiran, 1995). Bromocriptine was given initially at a dosage of 10 mg/day, and then 25 mg/day (no placebo). The main outcome measure was a stratified version of the Aphasia Test for Turkish Citizens where a speech sample was analysed and rated as either "A" (absence of speech), "B" (utterances with polymorphic syllabic fragments and phonemic jargon) or "C" (marked dysarthria and frequent stops within utterances). This outcome measure is almost certainly insensitive to the changes likely to be found with a drug therapy. Bromocriptine was found to be ineffective.

A further case report of similar design but with superior outcome measures was published as a book chapter (Berthier, 1999). This was an interesting case as the patient, who suffered bi-hemispheric, subcortical strokes 7 months apart, had Parkinsonian features as well as word-finding difficulties. After baseline assessment, there was a clear improvement in the amount of speech produced (53 words in 120 seconds of spoken picture description compared with six at baseline) with a more modest improvement (57 vs. 50) in confrontation naming. Some other test scores remained static suggesting some domain specificity, but with the lack of a placebo control, and thus any attempt at blinding, any effects beyond the clearly impressive motoric ones, are hard to interpret.

Gold, VanDam, and Silliman (2000) reported positive effects of bromocriptine in a small ($n = 4$, no placebo) trial of ABBA design (Gold, VanDam, & Silliman, 2000). Drug therapy was not paired with SALT. They specifically targeted anomia and used a bespoke anomia test with 420 items split into six lists of 70 matched items, (parallel forms), which were computer-delivered. Reaction times were measured and the authors also calculated a retrieval and storage quotient based on an analysis of error type. They found that all four subjects improved their retrieval quotients on the drug (with "large" effect sizes on Cohen's d (0.74–3.4)). These dropped back towards baseline once the drug was ramped down, in three out of the four subjects. If anything, the effect on storage was in the other direction (worse on drug) with no consistent effects on reaction times. There were no non-language tests.

Bragoni et al. (2000) used escalating doses of bromocriptine in 11 patients to reportedly good effect, but there were several major flaws. The study was placebo-controlled and tablet treatment was paired with SALT, but there was no block randomisation, so all the patients received placebo first and then bromocriptine (each block = 60 days). The authors claim the study was double-blinded, but it is not clear how the study design was concealed from the assessing therapists. Side effects were common with four patients dropping out because of these. Of the five that completed the study, three had nausea despite domperidone cover. Drug studies with a high incidence of side effects are likely to unblind subjects. Statistically significant improvements were seen in several language measures, but in all these analyses, the data following the drug and therapy block were compared with the baseline time point and not with the data collected after the placebo and therapy block, e.g. the two biggest effects were seen in reading aloud and dictation, but these improvements occurred after the placebo plus SALT block (26% and 43%, respectively) with only marginal improvement seen after the bromocriptine plus SALT block (29% and 47%, respectively). In short, despite the claims of the authors, the results do not so much advance the case of bromocriptine therapy as make a case for the effectiveness of SALT. Too great a dose of bromocriptine was used as side effects were prohibitively high.

In 2001, Raymer et al. (2001) used bromocriptine on a single-subject with transcortical motor aphasia due to a right frontal stroke. It was a no-placebo trial with an ABABA design. There was no mention of concomitant SALT. The authors included experimental (language) tasks that they predicted drug therapy would improve, and a control task (gesture), where they predicted no improvement. Multiple tests were carried out to establish a baseline and the main outcome was the slope (rate of improvement) in each of the four phases (the two drug blocks and the two following washout periods). The patient's ability to gesture did not improve significantly across any block. The biggest effect was on verbal fluency with the authors arguing that this was due to a bromocriptine as the rate of change on this measure was significant for the first drug block but not the baseline block or either of the washout blocks. However, the general trend in these control blocks was upwards and the appropriate comparison would have been to directly compare the slopes of the drug blocks with the control blocks, rather than comparing the slope of each block to the null (a flat line). In short, the study produced no convincing evidence of a drug effect.

All of the studies discussed so far had been carried out with patients suffering from post-stroke aphasia, but the next study was carried out on a group of six patients with primary progressive aphasia (Reed, Johnson, Thompson, Weintraub, & Mesulam, 2004). It is a short report of less than 400 words, so details are slim, but it appears to be a well-designed, placebo-controlled, double-blinded, crossover trial with three main outcome measures: naming, word fluency and narrative language. The blocks were ~12 weeks long and while all the patients declined over this period, there was a significant reduction in this decline for the bromocriptine block for the mean length of utterance score (part of the narrative language score), suggesting a beneficial effect of bromocriptine on the motoric aspects of speech.

The largest bromocriptine trial is the most recent one which included 38 patients (Ashtary, Janghorbani, Chitsaz, Reisi, & Bahrami, 2006). This study recruited subjects from a single site in Iran and was carried out in the acute phase. Subjects were randomised by coin toss into the placebo or drug group. Coin-tossing is not a recommended method for small trials as this can sometimes result in an allocation sequence leading to groups that differ, by chance, quite substantially in size or in the occurrence of prognostic factors (Altman & Bland, 1999); although that did not appear to be the case with this study. A low dose of bromocriptine (10 mg per day) was used and no side effects were reported. No mention was made whether concurrent SALT was received by the patients. Performance on seven language tests and a control task (gesture) was measured before and after therapy. The patients in both groups improved on all eight outcome measures with no significant differences between the two groups; that is, there were significant time effects but no significant drug vs. placebo effects.

The two most recent studies used L-dopa rather than bromocriptine. The first was a well-designed, two-group study in 39 patients in the acute phase, on average 5 weeks post-stroke. Tablet therapy was paired with SALT (Seniow, Litwin, Litwin, Lesniak, & Czlonkowska, 2009). L-dopa was used in a phasic manner, that is, 100 mg (Madopar 125) was given 30 min prior to a SALT session which lasted for 45 min and occurred five times a week for 3 weeks. Performance on 10 subtests of the Boston Diagnostic Aphasia Examination was measured before and after therapy. As with the Ashtary study, subjects in both groups improved significantly on all tests compared to baseline; however, there was a significant group (L-dopa > placebo) effect on confrontation naming and repetition. This seemed to be driven mainly by the patients with frontal lesions ($n = 12$). Unlike previous studies, no attempt was made to limit recruitment based on aphasia subtype.

The most recent study by Leeman et al. (2011) was also conducted in the acute phase ~7.5 weeks post-stroke and also used L-dopa in a phasic manner to augment SALT. The SALT therapy was more complex as it comprised of standard therapy in the afternoon, ~1 hour a day, with additional computer-assisted therapy in the mornings. This was a programme that presented pictures to patients which they had to name, but rather than name aloud, they had to type in the name of the item. The authors examined item-specificity of the trained items across each block. The study was a crossover one so each subject passed through drug and placebo blocks (block duration only 2 weeks). There was an impressive effect of the computerised therapy with naming accuracy improving on the trained list by 25% on average, but there was no interaction with drug/placebo block. Although the therapy was supposed to be timed with drug administration, it looks like some computerised sessions occurred in the afternoon. Given that the half-life of the active drug (L-dopa with benserazide) was 90 min, this may have led to under-dosing. The group was also small and mixed (three had head injury rather than stroke) although the crossover design should have helped reduce the effects of this somewhat. The authors' conclusions to their study pretty much mirror our general view that, "The type of substance, dose, time since brain injury and the type and intensity of therapy and timing between drug administration and therapy are important factors that need more systematic exploration (2011, p. 47)".

DISCUSSION

Of the 15 studies discussed here, only seven reported a positive effect of dopaminergic therapy. Two of these were randomised controlled trials, but the overall impression is that the balance of evidence suggests no beneficial effect, on average, across the studies. A rather out-of-date Cochrane review dismissed all the evidence from any of the dopaminergic therapy studies, although it was published prior to the more modern and more rigorously controlled studies (Greener, Enderby, & Whurr, 2001). In terms of the inferences one can make with frequentist statistics, positive studies carry more weight than negative studies. As Fisher said, after a negative study, one can only "withhold judgment" (Dienes, 2011); but negative studies are harder to publish and one can't help but wonder if publication bias is at work here, especially for the smaller, uncontrolled studies (Dwan et al., 2008).

If we put these concerns to one side for now and concentrate only on the positive studies, can we discern any pattern of improvement that may give a clue as to how and at what level (in terms of cognitive models) dopaminergic therapy may be working? Given that all of the studies focused either mainly or entirely on speech output, we can perhaps use Levelt's simplified model of speech production to try and assay where the positive effects are manifest. Levelt divides speech output into four main serial processes: concept generation, word-finding, motor planning and articulation (Levelt, 1999). In terms of which aspects of speech or language function improved, the following were found: naming/word-finding (5 studies); verbal fluency (which taps into several components of Levelt's model, 2 studies); motoric aspects of speech (repetition, 3 studies). Of course, this type of analysis is dependent on how often the individual measures were used and there is no accepted, standardised way of choosing outcomes in aphasia research. Almost all of the studies measured naming ability. There have been few studies in normal subjects that are relevant, but in a landmark study, Knecht and colleagues investigated the effect of L-dopa in normal subjects on novel word-learning in a randomised, placebo-controlled study (Knecht et al., 2004). They used 100 mg of L-dopa in a phasic manner, timed with computer-based learning of new words (pseudowords) for pictures of familiar items. The L-dopa group had significantly enhanced speed, overall success and long-term retention of novel word-learning than the placebo group, and they did so in a dose-dependent manner (while all subjects in the L-dopa group received the same dose, in a clever twist, the authors performed a subanalysis using a median split to assess this group by weight; the lighter subjects did significantly better). They included appropriate tests to rule out non-specific effects of motor performance, arousal, attention or response bias. The evidence from this study suggests that task-dependent learning can be improved by dopaminergic therapy, although the mechanism could be via the mesolimbic reward system (Fiorillo, Tobler, & Schultz, 2003), prefrontal cortical circuitry underlying working memory (Williams & Goldmanrakic, 1995) or via enhancing classical long-term potentiation at the hippocampal–prefrontal synapses (Gurden, Takita, & Jay, 2000). Returning to the patient data, it is very difficult to say much about the language specificity of these effects as few studies had a "control" outcome (two used gesture) where one might expect no effect of therapy. No studies reported measures of more basic cognitive components such as attention or vigilance which are likely to impact on any task-specific measures, which is a shame as there is good evidence that the dopaminergic system modulates these (Husain & Mehta, 2011); however, taken together with the Knecht study, the positive evidence points towards either new encoding (relearning) of word form information, or its enhanced retrieval as the most likely mechanism of action of dopaminergic therapy.

Perhaps the biggest surprise is the lack of agents tried. Bromocriptine dominates the literature, yet it has a poor side effect profile both in terms of short-term administration (as shown in several of the trials reviewed here that tried to push the dose to 30 mg/day and beyond) and in terms of longer-term risks of cardiorespiratory fibrosis. This agent would be unlikely to find many takers in real-world clinical practice. L-dopa has more translational potential but its bioavailability means that it is best suited for phasic use, perhaps paired with ongoing SALT. Both the trials using L-dopa were in the acute phase, but there is no good reason to think it would not work in the post-acute phase. Lastly, we were surprised that there are no studies with the newer dopaminergic agents. A search of the US and EU clinical trial databases revealed only a single ongoing trial of Tolcapone (a COMT inhibitor) in aphasic patients with fronto-temporal dementia. Perhaps future studies will consider the non-ergot-derived agonists or reuptake inhibitors such as methylphenidate.

All drug studies are resource-consuming and take a lot of effort, so what lessons can be learnt from the studies reviewed here that might guide future work? Perhaps firstly we should say that, given the effects and effect sizes of behavioural therapy, future studies should pair dopaminergic drug therapy with behavioural therapy of some sort; a view that others have endorsed (de Boissezon, Peran, de Boysson, & Demonet, 2007). While we can probably draw a veil over bromocriptine, it would be nice to see studies with newer agents or with L-dopa in the chronic phase. In terms of study design, generally, double-blind, randomised, placebo-controlled trials are best. Well-designed single-case or case-series studies are useful, but care should be taken to control for placebo and time effects, so multiple baseline, ramp-up, ramp-down or multiple alternating blocks (ABA, ABBA) should be considered (Hilliard, 1993). For group studies, we prefer crossover designs as these deal effectively with inter-subject variance, but if a more traditional two-group (or more) design is to be used, then block randomisation and/or minimisation should be employed to reduce the risk of the groups becoming unbalanced on key variables such as time since stroke or severity (Altman & Bland, 2005). Given the high incidence of side effects in some studies, building in a de-escalation option in the study protocol will help keep some patients in the study side effect-free, albeit on a lower dose. This seems reasonable as higher doses of cognitive enhancing drugs do not necessarily lead to better performance (Husain & Mehta, 2011). Studying patients in the acute phase, when "natural" recovery curves are at their steepest is always a challenge, but can be done using more innovative techniques such as randomised N-of-1 designs (Edgington & Onghena, 2007). Husain and colleagues used this in a study of the dopamine agonist rotigotine in acute, post-stroke neglect to good effect (Gorgoraptis et al., 2012). Finally, what to measure? It is probably not a good idea for language outcomes to be fixed for all aphasia studies, as these will need to be tailored to the impairments and disability profile of the participants, which will necessarily vary from study to study. Standardised tests that are sensitive to change, such as the Comprehensive Aphasia Battery (Swinburn, Porter, & Howard, 2004), are best. Non-language tests should also be included: probably a test of motor function (as the main function of dopamine is on the motor system) and also a test of attention. Lastly, patient-reported outcome measures should be used if possible because if we are to hope for clinical translation to proceed from clinical trials, we will need some evidence that patients or their carers find our interventions useful as well.

REFERENCES

Albert, M. L., Bachman, D. L., Morgan, A., & Helm-Estabrooks, N. (1988). Pharmacotherapy for aphasia. *Neurology, 38*, 877–879.

Alexander, G. E., DeLong, M. R., & Strick, P. L. (1986). Parallel organization of functionally segregated circuits linking basal ganglia and cortex. *Annual Review of Neuroscience, 9*, 357–381.

Allen, L., Mehta, S., McClure, J. A., & Teasell, R. (2012). Therapeutic interventions for aphasia initiated more than six months post stroke: A review of the evidence. *Top Stroke Rehabilitation, 19*, 523–535.

Altman, D. G., & Bland, J. M. (1999). Statistics notes – how to randomise. *British Medical Journal, 319*, 703–704.

Altman, D. G., & Bland, J. M. (2005). Treatment allocation by minimisation. *British Medical Journal, 330*, 843.

Andersohn, F., & Garbe, E. (2009). Cardiac and noncardiac fibrotic reactions caused by Ergot-and Nonergot-derived dopamine agonists. *Movement Disorders, 24*, 129–133.

Ashtary, F., Janghorbani, M., Chitsaz, A., Reisi, M., & Bahrami, A. (2006). A randomized, double-blind trial of bromocriptine efficacy in nonfluent aphasia after stroke. *Neurology, 66*, 914–916.

Benes, F. M. (2001). Carlsson and the discovery of dopamine. *Trends Pharmacoogical Sciences, 22*, 46–47.

Berthier, M. L. (1999). Transcortical motor aphasia. In M. L. Berthier (Ed.), *Transcortical aphasias* (37–74). Hove: Psychology Press.

Bragoni, M., Altieri, M., Di Piero, V., Padovani, A., Mostardini, C., & Lenzi, G. L. (2000). Bromocriptine and speech therapy in non-fluent chronic aphasia after stroke. *Neurological Sciences, 21*, 19–22.

Civelli, O., Bunzow, J. R., & Grandy, D. K. (1993). Molecular diversity of the dopamine receptors. *Annual Review of Pharmacology and Toxicology, 33*, 281–307.

de Boissezon, X., Peran, P., de Boysson, C., & Demonet, J. F. (2007). Pharmacotherapy of aphasia: Myth or reality? *Brain Language, 102*, 114–125.

Dienes, Z. (2011). Bayesian versus orthodox statistics: Which side are you on? *Perspectives on Psychological Science, 6*, 274–290.

Dwan, K., Altman, D. G., Arnaiz, J. A., Bloom, J., Chan, A. W., Cronin, E., . . . Williamson, P. R. (2008). Systematic review of the empirical evidence of study publication bias and outcome reporting bias. *PLoS ONE, 3*, e3081. doi:10.1371/journal.pone.0003081

Edgington, E., & Onghena, P. (2007). *Randomization tests (statistics: A series of textbooks and monographs)* (4th ed.). Boca Raton, FL: Chapman & Hall/CRC.

Fiorillo, C. D., Tobler, P. N., & Schultz, W. (2003). Discrete coding of reward probability and uncertainty by dopamine neurons. *Science, 299*, 1898–1902.

Goberman, A. M., & Coelho, C. (2002). Acoustic analysis of parkinsonian speech I: Speech characteristics and L-Dopa therapy. *NeuroRehabilitation, 17*, 237–246.

Gold, M., VanDam, D., & Silliman, E. R. (2000). An open-label trial of bromocriptine in nonfluent aphasia: A qualitative analysis of word storage and retrieval. *Brain Language*, *74*, 141–156.

Gorgoraptis, N., Mah, Y. H., Machner, B., Singh-Curry, V., Malhotra, P., Hadji-Michael, M., . . . Husain, M. (2012). The effects of the dopamine agonist rotigotine on hemispatial neglect following stroke. *Brain*, *135*, 2478–2491.

Gotham, A. M., Brown, R. G., & Marsden, C. D. (1988). Frontal cognitive function in patients with Parkinsons-disease on and off Levodopa. *Brain*, *111*, 299–321.

Greener, J., Enderby, P., & Whurr, R. (2001). Pharmacological treatment for aphasia following stroke. *Cochrane Database Systematic Review*, (4), CD000424. doi/10.1002/14651858.CD000424/abstract

Grossman, M., Glosser, G., Kalmanson, J., Morris, J., Stern, M. B., & Hurtig, H. I. (2001). Dopamine supports sentence comprehension in Parkinson's disease. *Journal of the Neurological Sciences*, *184*, 123–130.

Gupta, S. R., & Mlcoch, A. G. (1992). Bromocriptine treatment of nonfluent aphasia. *Archives of Physical Medicine and Rehabilitation*, *73*, 373–376.

Gupta, S. R., Mlcoch, A. G., Scolaro, C., & Moritz, T. (1995). Bromocriptine treatment of nonfluent aphasia. *Neurology*, *45*, 2170–2173.

Gurden, H., Takita, M., & Jay, T. M. (2000). Essential role of D1 but not D2 receptors in the NMDA receptor-dependent long-term potentiation at hippocampal-prefrontal cortex synapses in vivo. *Journal of Neuroscience*, *20*, RC106.

Hilliard, R. B. (1993). Single-case methodology in psychotherapy process and outcome research. *Journal of Consulting and Clinical Psychology*, *61*, 373–380.

Husain, M., & Mehta, M. A. (2011). Cognitive enhancement by drugs in health and disease. *Trends Cognitive Science*, *15*, 28–36.

Kertesz, A. (1982). *The western aphasia battery*. New York, NY: Grune and Stratton.

Knecht, S., Breitenstein, C., Bushuven, S., Wailke, S., Kamping, S., Floel, A., . . . Ringelstein, E. B. (2004). Levodopa: Faster and better word learning in normal humans. *Annals of Neurology*, *56*, 20–26.

Kvernmo, T., Hartter, S., & Burger, E. (2006). A review of the receptor-binding and pharmacokinetic properties of dopamine agonists. *Clinical Therapeurtics*, *28*, 1065–1078.

Lachin, J. M., Matts, J. P., & Wei, L. J. (1988). Randomization in clinical-trials – conclusions and recommendations. *Controlled Clinical Trials*, *9*, 365–374.

Lazar, R. M., Minzer, B., Antoniello, D., Festa, J. R., Krakauer, J. W., & Marshall, R. S. (2010). Improvement in aphasia scores after stroke is well predicted by initial severity. *Stroke*, *41*, 1485–1488.

Leemann, B., Laganaro, M., Chetelat-Mabillard, D., & Schnider, A. (2011). Crossover trial of subacute computerized aphasia therapy for anomia with the addition of either levodopa or placebo. *Neurorehabil Neural Repair*, *25*, 43–47.

Levelt, W. J. M. (1999). Models of word production. *Trends in Cognitive Neuroscience*, *3*, 223–232.

Lomas, J., & Kertesz, A. (1978). Patterns of spontaneous recovery in aphasic groups: A study of adult stroke patients. *Brain Language*, *5*, 388–401.

MacLennan, D. L., Nicholas, L. E., Morley, G. K., & Brookshire, R. H. (1991). The effects of bromocriptine on speech and language function in a patient with transcortical motor aphasia. In T. E. Prescott (Ed.), *Clinical Aphasiology* (Vol. 20). Boston, MA: College Hill.

Missale, C., Nash, S. R., Robinson, S. W., Jaber, M., & Caron, M. G. (1998). Dopamine receptors: From structure to function. *Physiogical Review*, *78*, 189–225.

Moss, A., & Nicholas, M. (2006). Language rehabilitation in chronic aphasia and time postonset: A review of single-subject data. *Stroke*, *37*, 3043–3051.

Ozeren, A., Sarica, Y., Mavi, H., & Demirkiran, M. (1995). Bromocriptine is ineffective in the treatment of chronic nonfluent aphasia. *Acta Neurologica Belgica*, *95*, 235–238.

Price, C. J., Seghier, M. L., & Leff, A. P. (2010). Predicting language outcome and recovery after stroke: The PLORAS system. *Nature Reviews Neurology*, *6*, 202–210.

Quaglieri, C. E., & Celesia, G. G. (1977). Effect of Thalamotomy and Levodopa therapy on speech of Parkinson patients. *European Neurology*, *15*, 34–39.

Raymer, A. M., Bandy, D., Adair, J. C., Schwartz, R. L., Williamson, D. J., Gonzalez Rothi, L. J., & Heilman, K. M. (2001). Effects of bromocriptine in a patient with crossed nonfluent aphasia: A case report. *Archives of Physical Medicine and Rehabilitation*, *82*, 139–144.

Reed, D. A., Johnson, N. A., Thompson, C., Weintraub, S., & Mesulam, M. M. (2004). A clinical trial of bromocriptine for treatment of primary progressive aphasia. *Annals of Neurology*, *56*, 750.

Sabe, L., Leiguarda, R., & Starkstein, S. E. (1992). An open-label trial of bromocriptine in nonfluent aphasia. *Neurology*, *42*, 1637–1638.

Sabe, L., Salvarezza, F., Garcia Cuerva, A., Leiguarda, R., & Starkstein, S. (1995). A randomized, double-blind, placebo-controlled study of bromocriptine in nonfluent aphasia. *Neurology*, *45*, 2272–2274.

Seniow, J., Litwin, M., Litwin, T., Lesniak, M., & Czlonkowska, A. (2009). New approach to the rehabilitation of post-stroke focal cognitive syndrome: Effect of levodopa combined with speech and language therapy on functional recovery from aphasia. *Journal of the Neurological Sciences*, *283*, 214–218.

Swinburn, K., Porter, G., & Howard, D. (2004). *Comprehensive Aphasia Test*. Hove: Psychology Press.

Williams, G. V., & Goldmanrakic, P. S. (1995). Modulation of memory fields by dopamine D1 receptors in prefrontal cortex. *Nature*, *376*, 572–575.

A clinical study of the combined use of bromocriptine and speech and language therapy in the treatment of a person with aphasia

Mandy A. Galling[1], Neetish Goorah[2], Marcelo L. Berthier[3], and Karen Sage[4]

[1]Speech and Language Therapy, East Lancashire Hospitals NHS Trust, Burnley, UK
[2]Stroke and Elderly Medicine, East Lancashire Hospitals NHS Trust, Burnley, UK
[3]Unit of Cognitive Neurology and Aphasia, Centro de Investigaciones Médico-Sanitarias (CIMES), University of Málaga, Málaga, Spain
[4]School of Psychological Sciences, University of Manchester, Manchester, UK

Background: Bromocriptine has been used in previous studies to treat people with non-fluent aphasia with varying levels of success.
Aims: This single case study set out to describe the effect of a 30 mg dose of bromocriptine on the behaviour, cognition and linguistic skills of a person with aphasia post-cerebrovascular accident.
Methods & Procedures: The participant received speech and language therapy alone and combined with the drug. Four testing points were made to examine the effects of bromocriptine: (1) at baseline before the drug was administered, (2) once the drug reached 30 mg dosage, (3) after the combined speech and language therapy and drug regime and (4) after drug and therapy withdrawal.
Outcomes & Results: The participant responded on all behavioural measures to the use of bromocriptine. The combined use of speech and language therapy with bromocriptine provided clear improvements in the participant's overall behaviours and specifically in her verbal output.
Conclusions: There is a case for the careful and correct selection of participants to use bromocriptine in combination with speech and language therapy. People who are adynamic, have non-fluent Broca's type or transcortical motor type aphasia may benefit from this combined treatment.

We are indebted to JS and her family for agreeing to take part in the study, their patience, their feedback and their insights into the study. Thanks also to Sian Davies, speech and language therapy manager, who encouraged and enabled this study. Thanks to Dr. Goorah's team and GP who helped in monitoring the participant's health and well-being during this study.

The use of drugs to enhance the rehabilitation of people post-cerebrovascular accident (CVA) has been explored over past decades, sometimes to lessen the effects of apathy (Jorge, Starkstein, & Robinson, 2010; Starkstein & Manes, 2000) but most commonly to alleviate depression (Jorge, Acion, Moser, Adams, & Robinson, 2010; Paolucci, 2008) which has been shown to be even more likely in people with aphasia (Kauhanen et al., 2000). For example, drug treatment for depression was high across four stroke rehabilitation settings in Switzerland (Englelter et al., 2012). However, in the same study, levodopa and acetylcholinesterase inhibitors were also used in people for whom their use was not clearly linked to the presenting symptoms (only two of the six people who were prescribed levodopa had symptoms linked with Parkinson's disease). No large scale randomised controlled trial (RCT) into the use of pharmaceutical interventions to enhance the uptake of therapy has taken place and, in the UK, there has been no licensing of any drug specifically to do this.

Drug treatment for people with aphasia has been built upon the assumption that stroke lesions disrupt neurotransmitter activity in the area of damage and also in dysfunctional neighbouring and remote regions in ipsilesional and contralesional hemispheres (Berthier & Pulvermüller, 2011; Gratton, Nomura, Pérez, & D'Esposito, 2012). The underlying assumption is that more functional brain activity might be regained by up-regulating or leveraging the activity of neurotransmitters (e.g., excessive glutamate release) in dysfunctional brain areas nearby or distant to the structurally damaged tissue. This might eventually lead to restored cognitive and behavioural functions. The anatomic distribution of neurotransmitter systems in the brain varies for each transmitter. Indeed, some neurotransmitters are present in virtually every part of the brain (e.g., glutamate, gamma-aminobutyric acid (GABA)) while others innervate relatively small cortical fields (e.g., acetylcholine, dopamine; Amunts et al., 2010; Berthier & Pulvermüller, 2011). Therefore, damage to some structures might predominantly deplete the activity of some neurotransmitters while having little impact on others. For example, the dopaminergic neural pathways emanate from the midbrain tiers (substantia nigra, pars compacta and ventral tegmental area) and ascend to innervate the basal ganglia and specific cortical sites (supplementary motor area, anterior cingulate and dorsolateral prefrontal and inferior parietal cortices). These neural pathways play a key role in controlling initiation and maintenance of complex motor routines, attention switching and goal-directed behaviour and motivation (Albert, Bachman, Morgan, & Helm-Estabrooks, 1988; Levy & Dubois, 2006). Damage to such regions can reduce the drive to generate speech (verbal adynamia), produce deficits in focusing attention and controlling cognition related to speech and language processes as well as decrease motivation (Alexander, 2006); all as a result of reduced availability of dopamine in the cerebral cortex and subcortical structures (Albert et al., 1988; Raymer, 2003). There is, therefore, an implicit expectation that enhancing dopaminergic activity with drugs may improve the cognitive and behavioural deficits which arise from this hypodopaminergic status. Dopaminergic drugs (levodopa, bromocriptine and rotigotine) have been used with variable results in the treatment of aphasia (Albert et al., 1988; Seniów, Litwin, Litwin, Leśniak, & Członkowska, 2009), neglect (Gorgoraptis et al., 2012) and motivational deficits (Powell, AlAdawi, Morgan, & Greenwood, 1996).

Since Albert et al.'s (1988) seminal description of the benefits of bromocriptine in a person with chronic transcortical motor aphasia, bromocriptine has been widely investigated in the treatment of aphasia (see Berthier, 2005 for a review).

Bromocriptine is a postsynaptic dopamine D2 receptor agonist and, in the UK, is prescribed in the management of Parkinson's disease (MIMS). It also has a role as a prolactine inhibitor to suppress lactation. Dopamine has several important roles including regulation of reward, attention, learning, mood and movement. The effects of bromocriptine use with people with aphasia have been variable (Berthier, 2005; Berthier, Pulvermüller, Dávila, García-Casares, & Gutiérrez, 2011). Of particular note for the present study were the positive effects seen in previous single case studies of transcortical motor aphasia, adynamic aphasia and Broca's aphasia (Albert et al., 1988; Berthier, 1999; Raymer, 2003; Raymer et al., 2001), where low/medium doses of bromocriptine (20–30 mg per day) were given and improvements in verbal fluency, response latency and confrontation naming tasks were observed. However, in those studies which reported longer term effects of the drug, gains made by participants in their verbal output were not maintained once the drug had been discontinued. Moreover, only two studies (Albert et al., 1988; Bragoni et al., 2000) combined specific speech and language treatment with the drug to explore its effect on the person's ability to benefit from therapy. Unfortunately, benefits reported in single case, case-series and open-label studies have not been replicated in RCTs (Ashtary, Janghorbani, Chitsaz, Reisi, & Bahrami, 2006; Sabe, Salvarezza, García Cuerva, Leiguarda, & Starkstein, 1995). There is also evidence that this drug is not suitable for all aphasia sub-types or for those with more severe aphasias (Gupta, Mlcoch, Scolaro, & Moritz, 1995). It stands to reason, therefore, that there needs to be strong theoretical reasons to provide a dopamine agonist to someone with aphasia and, to date, the profile which has shown most promise is that of "aphasic patients with selective impairments in energising attention and activating intended messages" (Berthier et al., 2011 p. 306). Optimal dosage, when the drug is used, has yet to be established (Berthier et al., 2011). Current evidence suggests that low to medium dosages (10–20 mg) are more likely to be successful with the right candidate, because such dosages are less likely to induce adverse events than higher doses (e.g., up to 60 mg per day).

This study will set out a single case study combining the use of bromocriptine alongside speech and language therapy in a person with aphasia. This person was selected because of her presentation to the rehabilitation team as adynamic, taking little part in rehabilitation tasks. Her aphasia profile showed some lack of initiation (in line with a profile of adynamic aphasia) (Costello & Warrington, 1986; Gold et al., 1997; Luria & Tsvetkova, 1968; Robinson, Blair, & Cipolotti, 1998), her spoken output resembled moderately severe Broca's type aphasia, though her repetition skills were slightly better than might be expected for such a profile and placed her on a continuum with transcortical aphasia (Berthier, 1999).

AIMS OF THIS STUDY

(1) To provide a close description of the participant's language, cognition and function and the clinical need to engage drug treatment.
(2) To find out whether bromocriptine drug therapy regime aiming to engage the dopamine pathways would have behavioural effects across World Health Organization (WHO, 2001) levels of impairment, activity and participation.
(3) To explore the reasons for choosing to combine drug and behavioural therapy.
(4) To look at the participant's response to the drug alone and the drug combined with impairment treatment.
(5) To examine whether skills were maintained when the drug was removed.

PARTICIPANT DESCRIPTION

Background biographical information

JS was a 58-year-old, right-handed, female at the time of her subarachnoid haemorrhage. She had a supportive partner and a large family of siblings, children and grandchildren. JS lived with her husband who worked full time. Prior to her subarachnoid haemorrhage, JS worked full time in a local café. JS' interests centred around her previous work and looking after the home. She had enjoyed bingo, crosswords and word searches. She used to meet and talk to people while she was at work but did not have a wide circle of friends. JS had been (and remained) a smoker with a history of raised blood pressure and diet-controlled diabetes. She was on hormone replacement therapy medication.

Onset and medical presentation and rehabilitation pathway

In 2005, JS suffered a subarachnoid haemorrhage secondary to the spontaneous rupture of a saccular aneurysm of the left internal carotid artery. An emergency computerised assisted tomography (CAT) scan before surgery (Figure 1a) showed a large, left frontal (orbital and medial cortices) and anterior temporal intracerebral haematoma, impinging on the ventral caudate nucleus and anterior hippocampus, with moderate lateral and third ventricle dilatation consistent with hydrocephalus. The aneurysm was successfully blocked with coiling and an extra-ventricular drain was inserted to control the hydrocephalus. A repeat CAT scan, taken 1 week after the endovascular procedure, showed a resolving left frontal haemorrhage (oedema persisted in the white matter close to the left dorsal caudate nucleus) together with a new, large area of infarction affecting the left temporo-parieto-occipital in the middle cerebral artery territory (Figure 1 a and b).

JS had a right-sided weakness with a more significant degree of impairment in the upper limb than the lower. She had problems sustaining attention. She had an aphasic language profile; her auditory comprehension was inconsistent beyond the single word level and her spoken output comprised social stereotypes only. There were no swallowing problems. JS returned home 2 months after the cerebral bleeding by which time she was able to walk independently with a stick. She required assistance to bathe or shower but was able to dress herself. Other family members took full responsibility for shopping, cooking and cleaning the house. Rehabilitation professionals described her as "subdued". In the kitchen, she had problems sequencing events correctly and could not find the equipment she needed. Her score on the Frenchay Aphasia Screening Test (FAST; Enderby, Wood, & Wade, 1987) at this time was 2/30 (a score gained from the comprehension section only as she did not score on the expressive section). Spoken and written comprehension of single words (as measured by Psycholinguistic Assessments of Language Processing in Aphasia (PALPA) 47 and 48; Kay, Lesser, & Coltheart, 1992) were also impaired (35/40 and 33/40, respectively). In January 2006, her Barthel index (Mahoney & Barthel, 1965) was 96/100 and rehabilitation professionals noted that she was "quiet but speaks when spoken to". The speech and language therapist (SLT) observed limited interaction with others at the day rehabilitation unit. She attended regularly but showed little enthusiasm for activities. She took little pride in her appearance. She was able to make a hot meal with support but could not correctly set cutlery on the table or use equipment such as scissors or tin openers. Language testing of naming, repetition and reading aloud was abandoned because of

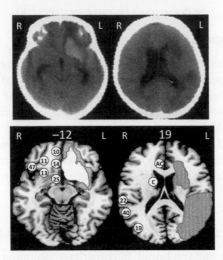

Figure 1. The upper panel shows axial slices of CAT scans carried out shortly after the subarachnoid haemorrhage (left image) and after endovascular coiling (right image). The left image shows a large parenchymal haemorrhage involving the left frontal basal and medial region surrounded by vasogenic oedema and mass effect causing a shift of midline structures and discrete ventricular compression. The right image shows a left anterior subcortical area of vasogenic oedema associated with the frontobasal haemorrhage (not shown) and an acute area of infarction in the left temporo-parieto-occipital junction. Also note (left and right images) ventricular dilatation consistent with mild communicating hydrocephalus. In the lower panel, the topography of lesions is drawn in axial images from the MRIcroN (http://www.mccauslandcenter.sc. edu/mricro/mricron/) at levels –12 and 19 together with the corresponding Brodmann's areas compromised by the lesions drawn in left side of the image. Brodmann's areas were selected using the BrainVoyager Brain Tutor (www.brainvoyager.com/BrainTutor.html). In the left image, the haemorrhage is depicted in white and perilesional oedema in grey, whereas in the right image areas of oedema (frontosubcortical) and the temporo-parieto-occipital infarction are shown in grey. Brodmann's areas affected by the left frontal lesion include 10, 11, 13, 14, 25 and head of the caudate nucleus and areas 22, 40 and 19 are affected by the temporo-parieto-occipital infarction. R indicates right; L indicates left; C indicates caudate and AC indicates anterior cingulum.

the level of distress this caused JS when she was required to access a specific word. However, at times, she was heard to use phrase level constructions. These were rare but fluently articulated. Phrase level output was more likely when JS was cross with somebody.

Impairment treatment prior to drug intervention

In February 2006, 4 months post-onset, her comprehension skills (for example, on measures such as PALPA 47 and 48; Kay et al., 1992) showed sufficient grasp of semantic concepts to suggest moving the focus of therapy away from this towards improving the continued paucity of specific expressive output. A core target vocabulary of 20 items was agreed with JS, comprising family names, places in the town where she lived, toiletry/household/clothing items. These were represented as pictures with the written word underneath. A combination of tasks was used with this vocabulary, including identifying the target from description, repetition of the word with picture and written cue, reading aloud with picture and written cue, copying a gesture modelled by the SLT, copying the written word, naming the item from the picture and written cue. This treatment protocol was carried out twice a week with the SLT, each session lasting between 30–45 min. During this time, her repetition skills improved but there was no change in reading aloud or naming. JS was able to reproduce actions which required a pointing response (e.g., pointing to shoes) but could not coordinate a sequence of movements to represent a symbolic gesture (e.g., rubbing hands to indicate hand cream). At this stage, a formal assessment of her output skills was made using PALPA 53 (Kay et al., 1992) which uses the same items to access spoken naming, written naming, reading aloud and repetition across modalities. She was unable to score on spoken and written naming or reading aloud but did score 33/40 on repetition. Although her repetition score was considerably better than other language skills, this score was more than two standard deviations below the control mean. In July 2006 (9 months post-onset), the treatment regime was adapted in case the lack of change was due to the method used. Twenty items were targeted which included 11 nouns from PALPA 53 (Kay et al., 1992) along with family names and personal vocabulary. The 11 PALPA nouns were included in order to assess whether treated items were benefitting from this adapted therapy. All items were represented as a picture with the written word below. Tasks included repetition of each item, producing the target from a lead-in phrase, e.g., "Your husband's name is . . . ?", naming the picture (if unsuccessful, JS was given the initial syllable cue or whole word cue to repeat), copy writing. This regime resulted in an improvement in repetition (18/20), naming cued by phrase (15/20) and confrontation naming (9/20). JS was able to name four of the untreated PALPA times following this treatment. Thus, although this change was not large, it did suggest the possibility of a shift in spoken naming. However, JS continued to appear passive and only attempted to offer verbal information when asked specific questions or when angry. She tended to wear the same clothes and remained dependent on her family for shopping, cooking and cleaning, even though she was physically much stronger, reflecting a possible action planning disorder. The SLT suspected that JS' lack of drive may have had an influence on the extent to which she was able to benefit from speech and language therapy and that the potential for change in her expressive output was not being maximised.

In people where there may be damage to dopaminergic pathways in the orbitofrontal, medial and dorsolateral prefrontal cortices, anterior cingulate gyrus or basal ganglia (e.g., caudate nucleus), the dopaminergic agonist bromocriptine might be helpful in boosting attention, responsiveness to environment, action planning, mood and motivation (Berthier, 1999). Consequently, this drug was considered for use in this case to encourage changes in JS' alertness; decrease her passivity, increase her engagement in tasks, reduce her overall adynamic features and specifically to improve her ability to actively engage in her therapy programme, thereby increasing her verbal output.

METHODS AND PROCEDURES

Drug procedure

Bromocriptine was introduced according to the drug specifications and under the auspices of the consultant physician. The consultant physician explained that this use of bromocriptine was outside its UK licence and it was prescribed as an off-label drug (a medication to treat a condition before that use has been approved by the regulatory agencies). He provided oral and written information and explanation to both the participant and her partner as to why the drug might be of use and possible side effects.

TABLE 1
Linguistic and cognitive assessments linked with JS' drug regime

Week	0	1–4	5	6–8	9	13–15	16	17–41	50	51	52–62	63–86
mg daily	0	1.5–7.5	10	12.5–17.5	20	22.5–27.5	30	30	30	30		0
SLT intervention	No	No	No	No	No	No	No	Yes	Yes	No	No	No
Cognitive tests	x						x				Washout 5 mg	x (86)
WAB	x		x				x		x			x (86)
Cookie theft	x						x			x	every 4 weeks	
PALPA 53	x						x			x		

Western Aphasia Battery (WAB; Kertesz, 2007); Cookie theft picture (Goodglass et al., 2001); Psycholinguistic Assessments of Language Processing in Aphasia (PALPA; Kay et al., 1992).

JS and her husband then considered the information and agreed to its use. JS was reviewed in the consultant clinic every 4 weeks for the first 16 weeks (first 4 months). During the introduction and dose titration of the drug (weeks 1–16, see Table 1) no therapy was given by the SLT, though she visited weekly to check if there had been any side effects and to alert and liaise with the consultant if required. The family also had telephone contact details for the consultant should there be any emergency or other concern outside of normal clinic hours. Neither of these alerts was required. The bromocriptine was introduced gradually starting at 1.5 mg and increasing in 2.5 mg steps weekly (see Table 1) until a daily dose of 20 mg was reached. JS stayed on a daily dose of 20 mg for 4 weeks until the dose was again increased in 2.5 mg steps to 30 mg dose. Once JS achieved a dose of 30 mg daily, the gap between consultant checks was increased to 2 months, then 3 and then settled into 6 monthly reviews. Table 1 sets out the drug regime, the dosage increases and the timing of the assessments and of the speech and language intervention in weeks.

Local National Health Service (NHS) ethical approval was provided to study the effects of the behavioural treatment. Prior to the introduction of the drug, JS underwent a series of cognitive and linguistic tests to enable a description of her skills and deficits.

Assessment and outcome measure protocol

Assessments of cognitive skills (assessments 1–3) and aphasia (assessments 4–6) were completed before the drug procedure was introduced (see Table 1). The complete set of assessments used was:

(1) Test of Everyday Attention (TEA; Robertson, Ward, Ridgeway, & Nimmo-Smith, 1994) map search and elevator counting in sustained and divided conditions. The map search is a visual attention task in which the participant looks for a symbol on a map (e.g., petrol station symbol). The number of items identified in 1 min and after 2 minutes searching is scored. The elevator counting is an auditory attention task in two parts. In the sustained attention task, the participant hears a number of beeps and counts these in order to identify which floor the elevator (lift) has reached. In the divided attention task, the participant is required to do the same task but this time has to ignore the lower-toned beeps which are interspersed with the "elevator" beeps.

(2) Coloured Progressive Matrices (Raven, 1976) is a non-verbal reasoning task which requires the participant to select, from a choice of six, a missing piece to make up a pattern. The total score (36) is derived from the number of matrices completed correctly.

(3) Trail Making Test (TMT; Lezak et al., 2011; Reitan, 1958) is a pen and paper task composed of two parts (A and B). Both parts of the TMT consist of 25 circles distributed over a sheet of paper. In Part A, the circles are numbered 1–25 and the participant draws lines to connect the numbers in ascending order. In Part B, the task includes both numbers (1–13) and letters (A–L). As in Part A, the participant draws lines to connect the circles in an ascending pattern but with the added difficulty of alternating between the numbers and letters (e.g., 1-A; 2-B; 3-C). This assessment is timed.

(4) PALPA 53 (Kay et al., 1992) is an assessment of word retrieval for 40 high frequency picture items, across 5 different modalities (spoken naming, written naming, repetition, reading aloud and writing to dictation). JS was asked to provide a spoken name, written name, repeat and read aloud the 40 items.

(5) The Cookie theft picture from the Boston Diagnostic Aphasia Examination (Goodglass, Kaplan, & Barresi, 2001) allows the participant with aphasia to provide a verbal description of what is happening in the picture and provides some linguistic information about their verbal skills beyond single word naming.

(6) Western Aphasia Battery (WAB; Kertesz, 2007). The language components of the battery include spontaneous speech (fluency and information content), auditory comprehension, repetition, naming, reading and writing. The battery explores language levels in increasing complexity across single word, sentence and paragraph. An aphasia quotient (AQ) is calculated from the oral language tests (excluding the reading scores) and is a global measure of aphasia severity which has previously been sensitive enough to detect longitudinal changes in drug trials (Berthier et al., 2011).

Interim assessment to monitor the drug's effect was made using the WAB (Kertesz, 2007) and Cookie theft picture description (Goodglass et al., 2001). These were completed when the drug dose reached 10 mg and 20 mg. The complete set of assessments was repeated when the drug dose reached 30 mg (see Table 1).

Impairment intervention procedure

Speech and language therapy: Stage 1. This treatment began when the drug dose reached 30 mg and after the second set of full assessments had been completed. A 34 item vocabulary set was generated using 20 items from PALPA 53 (Kay et al., 1992) and 14 personally relevant names chosen by JS and her family. Each item was represented as a picture with the written word below. One treatment visit of around 45 min duration was provided weekly. At each visit, JS and the therapist undertook the programme set out below for each of the 34 items; all 5 steps were provided per item before moving onto the next item:

(1) The picture with written word was shown to JS and the SLT said the word for her to repeat.

(2) The picture was shown again and the SLT gave an initial syllable cue. If this did not prompt the correct word, then the SLT gave the whole word for repetition.

(3) The picture was shown again and the SLT gave an initial phoneme cue. If this did not prompt the correct word, then the initial syllable cue was tried. If this was not sufficient then the whole word was supplied for repetition.

(4) A phrase was supplied to cue the picture name, e.g., "Your husband's name is . . .?"

(5) Uncued production of the name from the picture with written word.

Speech and language therapy: Stage 2. After 12 weeks, the treatment was altered by removing the written word from the pictures. The vocabulary was elicited using picture only and word only materials using the same cueing hierarchy:

(1) Say the word from an initial syllable cue.
(2) Say the word from an initial phoneme cue.
(3) Say the word with no additional cue.

This pattern of treatment was delivered in one visit per week for 45 min for another 12 weeks.

Speech and language therapy: Stage 3. A picture cue with a written label was produced for a number of nouns, verbs and adjectives which could be combined to build sensible clauses. At each session, JS was required to look at the picture with written word and:

(1) Repeat the single words.
(2) Repeat the same words in combination (e.g., noun with verb).
(3) Read aloud the single words.
(4) Read aloud in combination.
(5) Read aloud the same clauses with the picture removed.
(6) Describe the pictured clauses with the written cue removed.

This treatment was continued for 8 weeks.

Washout. At the end of these stages of treatment, a phased reduction in the dose of bromocriptine was planned. This was managed pragmatically so that, if JS, her treating therapist or physician felt that there was a decline in her abilities, there was an option to return to the dose level which had been therapeutic for her. No SLT was provided during the washout phase but review assessments (naming and reading aloud) from PALPA (Kay et al., 1992) were completed every 4 weeks to detect any signs of decline. The dose of bromocriptine was reduced by 5 mg every 4 weeks until she reached a dose of 5 mg. JS remained on 5 mg for 2 weeks and then the drug was removed altogether.

The TEA visual and auditory subtests (Robertson et al., 1994), the WAB (Kertesz, 2007) and Coloured Progressive Matrices (Raven, 1976) were repeated after 6 months without bromocriptine.

RESULTS

Drug procedure

Use of bromocriptine was safe and well tolerated at all doses. JS reported a reduction in her appetite but weight checks showed she had gained weight.

Measurement of effects of combined drug and speech and language therapy

Behaviour. In the early stages, there was no discernible change in behaviour. However, as the dose progressed to 20 mg and beyond, JS appeared to be taking more care with her appearance; she washed her hair more often and was wearing clothes in different styles. She telephoned the SLT department herself to rearrange appointments and informed the SLT if she was due to be reviewed by the consultant. She started doing more cooking. JS also reported more dissatisfaction and frustration with her limits in conversation and that she was missing work and the people she used to meet there. Overall, JS, her family and consultant were pleased with her progress and felt that there were changes in her communication at home; she was motivated to go out and she had drive to complete tasks around the home which made a difference to her quality of life. She and her husband held a party to celebrate an anniversary and she visited her sister in another county when that sister became unwell. These examples of everyday social interaction are ones she would not have confidently undertaken before the drug was provided.

Cognitive changes (Table 2). The scores on the TMT showed a decrease in the number of errors and an increase in speed of completion for both simple (Part A) and complex (Part B) trials. At baseline, the task was completed in a speed outside normal limits and was littered with errors. At a dose of 30 mg, JS completed the task accurately but her speed remained outside normal limits. Accuracy was maintained and speed of completion moved to within normal limits when she was retested after speech and language therapy treatment combined with 30 mg of bromocriptine and after the washout period. The sustained attention condition of the elevator counting on the TEA (Robertson et al., 1994) was borderline impaired at baseline (score of 6). This score improved to 7 (within normal limits) at a dose of 30 mg and after washout.

Changes on aphasia assessments (Table 3). At baseline, the AQ of the WAB (Kertesz, 2007) was 22.0 with a rating of very severe aphasia. This improved to 35.3 with severe aphasia by the end of treatment and drug washout. This improvement represents an increase in AQ–WAB score of 13.5 points). Cookie theft transcriptions (Goodglass et al., 2001) showed a gradual increase in the amount of information

TABLE 2
JS' scores on the cognitive assessments over time, linked to drug regime

	Week	0	5	9	16	17–41	51–62	86	No of items
	mg daily	0	10	20	30	30& SLT	Washout	0	
TEA map	1 min	10			17			19	77
	2 min	21			33			38	
TEA elevator	Sustained	6			7			7	7
	Divided	5			8			6	10
	Coloured Progressive Matrices	26			26			30	36
Trail making	Simple	120 sec*			132 sec ˆ			**75 sec** ˆ	
	Complex	270 sec*			305 sec ˆ			**132 sec** ˆ	

Test of Everyday Attention (TEA; Robertson et al., 1994); Trail Making Test (TMT; Reitan, 1958); Coloured Progressive Matrices (RCPM; Raven, 1976). Bold = within normal range, * errorful completion of the task; ˆ correct completion of the task.

TABLE 3
JS' scores on linguistic assessments over time, linked to drug regime

	Week	0	5	9	16	17–41	50	51	86	Max
	mg daily	0	10	20	30	30 +SLT	30 +SLT	30	0	
WAB Subtest scores	Aphasia raw score	22.0	24.8	28.8	31.1				35.3	
	Aphasia quotient*	43.9	49.6	57.6	62.2				70.6	
	Spontaneous speech (raw)	7	9	12	14				14	20
	Comprehension (÷ 20)	8.6	8.6	9.4	9.4				8.7	10
	Repetition (÷10)	3.0	2.7	2.7	2.8				5.0	10
	Naming (÷10)	3.3	4.5	4.7	4.9				7.6	10
	Reading and writing (raw)	58	66	124	125				110	200
PALPA 53	Spoken naming	13			12		20	31		40
	Reading aloud	10			–		32	37		40
	Repetition	37			**39**		**39**	–		40

Western Aphasia Battery (WAB; Kertesz, 2007); Psycholinguistic Assessments of Language Processing in Aphasia (PALPA; Kay et al., 1992);
Bold = within normal range.
* AQ is calculated by adding spontaneous speech raw score, comprehension score ÷ 20, repetition score ÷ 10 and naming score ÷ 10. Total is then multiplied by 2 to give aphasia quotient.
(For aphasia severity ratings and aphasia sub-types, see Kertesz, 2007.)

conveyed as the dose of bromocriptine increased (see Appendix A). At baseline, information content was poor and JS used pointing to the picture as an adjunct to her spoken description which contained three utterances. At a dose of 30 mg, JS did not need to point to the picture. There was an increase in the number of verb tokens used (from two to seven) over eight utterances. At the end of SLT intervention with a 30 mg dose of bromocriptine, JS was using longer and more complex utterances as well as conjunctions. A total of seven utterances were used (three using a conjunction) with nine verb tokens. A similar pattern was shown in the scoring of her spontaneous speech in the WAB (Kertesz, 2007). Comprehension subtests on the WAB showed little change. Spoken naming on PALPA 53 (Kay et al., 1992) did not show any change as the dose of bromocriptine increased (12/40). There was an improvement to 20/40 at the end of the SLT intervention (with the 30 mg bromocriptine dose). This score improved further to 31/40 as naming was monitored during the drug washout phase (all differences' significant using one-tailed McNemar test; 12/40 to 20/40; $p = .038$; 12/40 to 31/40, $p < .001$; 20/40 to 31/40, $p < .005$). JS scored 10/40 in reading aloud at baseline. At the end of the SLT intervention with 30 mg bromocriptine, there had been a significant improvement to 32/40 (McNemar, one-tailed, $p < .0001$). There was a further increase to 37/40 over the drug washout phase (difference from baseline to washout, McNemar, one-tailed, $p < .0001$, from end of intervention to washout, McNemar, one-tailed, $p = .056$). JS scored 37/40 in repetition at baseline. This improved to a near ceiling score of 39/40 once she reached 30 mg bromocriptine dose, prior to SLT treatment and she retained this score after the SLT intervention with the bromocriptine. JS' naming score on the WAB (Kertesz, 2007) improved significantly from 33/100 at baseline to 49/100 with a 30 mg dose of bromocriptine, prior to therapy (McNemar, one-tailed, $p = .035$). This improvement continued to 76/100 when reassessed 6 months after removing the bromocriptine (baseline to post-intervention and 30 mg to post-intervention, both McNemar, one-tailed, $p < .0001$). Repetition did not change from baseline to 30 mg dose (28/100) but there was a significant improvement to 50/100 after 6 months with no bromocriptine (McNemar, one-tailed, $p < .0001$). Reading and writing scores improved from 58/200 to 125/200 when the dose reached 30 mg though this difference was not statistically different (McNemar, one-tailed, $p = .063$). This improvement was not maintained after the bromocriptine was removed going down to 110/200, though this score was higher than her baseline starting point.

DISCUSSION

The single case study was able to document skills and deficits in behaviour, cognition and language over time in order to explore the effect of speech and language therapy alone, the effect of bromocriptine alone and what happens when the two are combined. Previously, JS had shown a limited response to SLT aimed at improving her verbal output, in spite of an indication of her improvement in scores on semantic processing assessments. A lack of drive (apathy) was evident in her non-verbal behaviour and this was suspected to have an influence on her ability to learn and make progress during SLT treatment. The addition of bromocriptine showed some improvements to baseline scores of language and cognition but the most significant changes were seen when bromocriptine was combined with SLT. This combined approach enabled JS to engage in her environment, retain and build on gains in language tasks and to make noticeable progress with spoken output, not just on test scores but also in her everyday life. This progress was maintained when the bromocriptine was removed. Increases in her AQ–WAB (Kertesz, 2007) indicate that, although she still had a severe aphasia, she had made significant improvements in her language performance on that test. Greater improvements in AQs are usually expected in people who are more severely affected, because there is more room for improvement than in those who are mildly impaired where there are limited opportunities for measuring improvements because of ceiling effects (Kertesz, 1997). The evolution of JS' language profile after the combined treatment aligns with this pattern. Ramsberger and Marie (2007) suggest that when improvements in the language function of someone with moderate-to-severe aphasia are greater than 20%, such gains should be considered clinically relevant. Using these criteria, JS' improvement of 63.4% on the WAB–AQ after drug and behavioural interventions might be considered clinically relevant. What underlies the success of this case study may be the combination of selecting the right participant and finding the correct dosage for that participant, both factors considered important in the successful use of bromocriptine (Berthier et al., 2011). JS had non-fluent aphasia and was adynamic in her everyday behaviours. This profile, also shown in previous studies (Costello & Warrington, 1986; Gold et al., 1997), may be a key consideration when selecting potential people with aphasia who might respond to this drug regime (e.g., Albert et al., 1988; Raymer et al., 2001). The ability to maintain her skills once the drug had been withdrawn differs from other case histories and may be linked to the combination of drug and SLT intervention. It is possible that combining SLT with bromocriptine treatment may not only have boosted recovery but also consolidated gains even after drug withdrawal, perhaps by promoting lasting neuroplastic changes in dopaminergic pathways (Knecht et al., 2004). However, further studies in which similar aphasia sub-types are recruited would be required to confirm this. A more in-depth study of the dosage necessary to effect these changes is also needed as is an examination of whether other drugs which modulate the dopaminergic pathways (e.g., levodopa, rotigotine, ropirinole) might be more or less useful, provide different patterns of skill learning and impact differentially on behavioural deficits. Recent drug trials using levodopa have shown divergent results which were most likely contingent on differences in the studied samples. A double-blind placebo-controlled trial RCT of levodopa in combination with SLT reported greater benefits in verbal fluency and repetition in people with chronic aphasia treated with levodopa than with placebo and gains were associated with frontal lobe involvement (Seniów et al., 2009). In contrast, intensive computerised aphasia therapy for anomia combined with levodopa during 2 weeks provided no superior effect than placebo in people with subacute vascular or traumatic aphasias affecting mainly temporal and temporo-parietal regions (Leemann, Laganaro, Chetelat-Mabillard, & Schnider, 2011). A further RCT combining levodopa with SLT is ongoing (ClinicalTrials.gov Identifier: NCT01429077), but further studies are needed.

Brain imaging in JS identified two large left hemisphere lesions (frontal haemorrhage and temporo-parieto-occipital infarct). In keeping with previous trials of dopaminergic stimulation in aphasia (see Seniów et al., 2009) bromocriptine in JS exerted its beneficial effects on functions dependent upon dopaminergic activity in fronto-subcortical regions with little impact on other cognitive deficits (auditory comprehension, naming) ascribed to posterior cortical dysfunction on which dopaminergic stimulation is presumably less beneficial (Albert et al., 1988; Leemann et al., 2011; Seniów et al., 2009). Neuroimaging studies examining functional plasticity after aphasia therapy have revealed that recovery may rely on the function of non-language areas underpinning memory, attention processes and multimodal integration (see Menke et al., 2009). The left basal and medial frontal areas (Brodmann's areas (BA) 10, 11, 13, 14, 25) responsible for adynamia and related production deficits in JS do not belong to the core perisylvian region devoted to traditional linguistic processes (phonology, lexical-semantics). These cortical areas nevertheless may be components of neural networks contributing to the generation of verbal messages by igniting communication (Willems & Varley, 2010), facilitating word selection and initiation of speech (Crosson et al., 2005) and increasing alertness and energising mood (Johansen-Berg et al., 2008; Mayberg et al., 2005). A fluid orchestration of these cognitive and behavioural functions is needed for the engagement and maintenance of communication in response to internally generated or environmentally driven relevant stimuli. Therefore, extensive damage to such areas in JS can explain not only expressive, attentional, executive and behavioural deficits but might also account for the poor response to SLT alone because these lesioned areas could not participate in recovery processes. What remains to be explained, in the case of JS, is how treatment with bromocriptine alone and combined with SLT improved cognitive and behavioural performance dependent upon dopaminergic activity in the face of extensive left frontal damage. A control CAT scan (Figure 1b) revealed reduction of the left frontal haemorrhage, oedema and pressure effects over medial prefrontal cortex, suprarhinal cortex, subgenual cingulate cortex and ventral caudate. Therefore, it is possible that, once these structures had been released from pressure effects, they were able to be innervated by the mesocortical dopaminergic system, thus regaining some activity. Activity of these networks was not strong enough to promote recovery after SLT or bromocriptine alone but SLT in combination with bromocriptine may have boosted recovery through activity-dependent strengthening of task-relevant dopaminergic synapses (Knecht et al., 2004). Another, complimentary explanation might be that the beneficial effects of bromocriptine alone and paired with SLT additionally recruited activity of right frontal networks. Two lines of brain imaging evidence concur with this hypothesis. Crosson et al. (2005) used a word production paradigm (category-member generation) and functional magnetic resonance imaging (fMRI) in a participant (case X030) with residual non-fluent aphasia and left frontal lobe damage, sparing the basal ganglia before and after intention treatment. Intention refers to the selection of one action among several competing possibilities for execution and initiation of that action (Crosson et al., 2007). Intention treatment uses complex left-hand movements to initiate picture naming with the aim of recruiting the right frontal cortex (see Crosson et al., 2007 for further details). At baseline fMRI activation predominated in the right frontal lobe (lateral and medial), right thalamus and right caudate nucleus and this hemispheric reorganisation continued after intention treatment although activation in the right lateral and medial frontal lobe decreased, together with increased recruitment of right dorsal caudate and left basal ganglia. In an earlier study by Crosson et al. (2005), manipulation of intention was beneficial even when unpaired with drug treatment. Although a different SLT approach was used in JS, it might be argued that combined treatment in JS may have triggered a similar transfer of activity from left frontal lobe to right fronto-subcortical networks. In addition, Berthier (2012) found increased metabolic activity in people with chronic aphasia with left perisylvian damage who were treated with a combination of the cholinesterase inhibitor dopenezil and constraint-induced aphasia therapy. These increases correlated with gains in verbal production (bilateral BA 47 and 25, and left BA 11, 37, subthalamic nucleus and thalamus) and motivation (right BA 11, 13, 25, 47 and left BA 37). Although bromocriptine and donepezil target different neurotransmitter systems, acetylcholine-dopamine interactions exist (Lester, Rogers, & Blaha, 2010; Mark, Shabani, Dobbs, & Hansen, 2011) and each drug has independently shown beneficial effects on apathy (Marin, Fogel, Hawkins, Duffy, & Krupp, 1995; Whyte et al., 2008).

The present findings should be interpreted in the light of some methodological limitations. This was a clinical study carried out in the course of a busy clinical caseload and so the choice of measures as well as when and how often these were carried out, was limited by considerations of clinical practice and practicalities. In particular, a linguistic measure (such as the AQ) measured in week 51 (immediately after therapy and full dose bromocriptine) would have allowed a clearer separation of the necessary ingredients for change in this case and allowed a differentiation between effects of therapy and drug combined, separate from the drug alone during and after the washout period. The important changes in JS' behaviour were visible to the team, family and JS herself. However, an independent ADL and activity level (WHO, 2001) measure, carried out at regular intervals would have provided useful corroborative evidence to back up those observations. It is, after all, the aim of any rehabilitation team that gains in assessment scores transfer into activities of daily living. The study is, yet again, a single case and one which is an unusual presentation. The need for further amassing of robust evidence of who may and may not benefit from this kind of combined intervention, is still required and will necessitate similarly detailed descriptions of the individuals involved. This necessity is sometimes in conflict with the need for larger scale drug trials (Ashtary et al., 2006; Sabe et al., 1995) and the desire for uniform application of therapies which inevitably vary across individuals and therefore dilute any real effects which may be occurring (Bowen et al., 2012).

REFERENCES

Albert, M. L., Bachman, D. L., Morgan, A., & Helm-Estabrooks, N. (1988). Pharmacotherapy for aphasia. *Neurology*, *38*, 877–879.

Alexander, M. P. (2006). Impairments for procedures for implementing complex language are due to disruption of frontal attention processes. *Journal of the International Neuropsychological Society*, *12*, 236–247.

Amunts, K., Lenzen, M., Friederici, A. D., Schleicher, A., Morosan, P., Palomero-Gallagher, N., & Zilles, K. (2010). Broca's region: Novel organizational principles and multiple receptor mapping. *PLoS Biology*, *8*, e1000489.

Ashtary, F., Janghorbani, M., Chitsaz, A., Reisi, M., & Bahrami, A. (2006). A randomized, double-blind trial of bromocriptine efficacy in nonfluent aphasia after stroke. *Neurology*, *66*, 914–916.

Berthier, M. L. (1999). *Transcortical Aphasias*. Hove: Psychology Press.

Berthier, M. L. (2005). Poststroke aphasia. Epidemiology, pathophysiology and treatment. *Drugs & Aging*, *22*, 163–182.

Berthier, M. L. (2012). *Pharmacological interventions boost language and communication treatment effects in chronic post-stroke aphasia* (p. 23). Presented in the symposium Fortschritte in Neurowissenschaft und Neurorehabilitation der Sprache. 85. Kongress der Deutschen Gesellschaft für Neurologie mit Fortbildungsakademie. Hamburg. Hauptprogramm.

Berthier, M. L., & Pulvermüller, F. (2011). Neuroscience insights improve neurorehabilitation of poststroke aphasia. *Nature Review Neurology*, *7*, 86–97.

Berthier, M. L., Pulvermüller, F., Dávila, G., García-Casares, N., & Gutiérrez, A. (2011). Drug therapy of post-stroke aphasia: A review of current evidence. *Neuropsychology Review*, *21*, 302–317.

Bowen, A., Hesketh, A., Patchick, E., Young, A., Davies, L., Vail, A., . . . Tyrell, P. (2012). Effectiveness of enhanced communication therapy in the first four months after stroke for aphasia and dysarthria: A randomised controlled trial. *British Medical Journal*, *345*, e4407.

Bragoni, M., Altieri, M., Di Piero, V., Padovani, A., Mostardini, C., & Lenzi, G. L. (2000). Bromocriptine and speech therapy in non-fluent chronic aphasia after stroke. *Neurological Sciences*, *21*, 19–22.

Bromocriptine in MIMS. Retrieved from http://www.mims.co.uk/.

Costello, A. L., & Warrington, E. W. (1986). Dynamic aphasia: The selective impairment of verbal planning. *Cortex*, *25*, 103–114.

Crosson, B., Bacon Moore, A., Gopinath, K., White, K. D., Wierenga, C. E., Gaiefsky, M. E., . . . Gonzalez Rothi, L. J. (2005). Role of the right and left hemispheres in recovery of function during treatment of intention in aphasia. *Journal of Cognitive Neuroscience*, *17*, 392–406.

Crosson, B., Fabrizio, K. S., Singletary, F., Cato, M. A., Wierenga, C. E., Parkinson, R. B., . . . Gonzalez Rothi, L. J. (2007). Treatment of naming in nonfluent aphasia through manipulation of intention and attention: A phase 1 comparison of two novel treatments. *Journal of the International Neuropsychological Society*, *13*, 582–594.

Enderby, P., Wood, V., & Wade, D. (1987). *Frenchay Aphasia Screening Test (FAST)*. Windsor: NFER-NELSON.

Engelter, S. T., Urscheler, N., Baronti, F., Vuadens, P., Koch, J., Frank, M., . . . Jenni, W. (2012). Frequency and determinants of using pharmacological enhancement in the clinical practice of in-hospital stroke rehabilitation. *European Neurology*, *68*, 28–33.

Gold, M., Nadeau, S. E., Jacobs, D. H., Adair, J. C., Gonzalez Rothi, L., & Heilman, K. M. (1997). Adynamic aphasia: A transcortical motor aphasia with defective semantic strategy formation. *Brain and Language*, *57*, 374–393.

Goodglass, H., Kaplan, E., & Barresi, B. (2001). *BDAE-3: The Boston diagnostic aphasia examination* (3rd ed.). Philadelphia, PA: Lippincott, Williams & Wilkins.

Gorgoraptis, N., Mah, Y. H., Machner, B., Singh-Curry, V., Malhotra, P., Hadji-Michael, M., . . . Husain, M. (2012). The effects of the dopamine agonist rotigotine on hemispatial neglect following stroke. *Brain*, *135*, 2478–2491.

Gratton, C., Nomura, E. M., Pérez, F., & D'Esposito, M. (2012). Focal brain lesions to critical locations cause widespread disruption of the modular organization of the brain. *Journal of Cognitive Neuroscience*, *24*, 1275–1285.

Gupta, S. R., Mlcoch, A. G., Scolaro, C., & Moritz, T. (1995). Bromocriptine treatment of nonfluent aphasia. *Neurology*, *45*, 2170–2173.

Johansen-Berg, H., Gutman, D. A., Behrens, T. E. J., Matthews, P. M., Rushworth, M. F. S., Katz, E., . . . Mayberg, H. S. (2008). Anatomical connectivity of the subgenual cingulate region targeted with deep brain stimulation for treatment-resistant depression. *Cerebral Cortex*, *18*, 1374–1383.

Jorge, R. E., Acion, L., Moser, D., Adams Jr, H. P., & Robinson, R. G. (2010). Escitalopram and enhancement of cognitive recovery following stroke. *Archives of general psychiatry*, *67*, 187–196.

Jorge, R. E., Starkstein, S. E., & Robinson, R. G. (2010). Apathy following stroke. *Canadian Journal of Psychiatry*, *55*, 350–354.

Kauhanen, M. L., Korpelainen, J. T., Hiltunen, P., Maatta, R., Mononen, H., Brusin, E., . . . Myllylä, V. V. (2000). Aphasia, depression, and non-verbal cognitive impairment in ischaemic stroke. *Cerebrovascular Diseases*, *10*, 455–461.

Kay, J., Lesser, R., & Coltheart, M. (1992). *Psycholinguistic Assessments of Language Processing in Aphasia (PALPA)*. Hove: Erlbaum.

Kertesz, A. (1997). Recovery of aphasia. In T. E. Feinberg & M. J. Farah (Eds.), *Behavioral neurology and neuropsychology*. New York, NY: McGraw-Hill.

Kertesz, A. (2007). *Western aphasia battery: Revised*. San Antonio, TX: Psychological Corporation.

Knecht, S., Breitenstein, C., Bushuven, S., Wailke, S., Kamping, S., Flöel, A., . . . Bernd Ringelstein, E. (2004). Levodopa: Faster and better word learning in normal humans. *Annals of Neurology*, *56*, 20–26.

Leemann, B., Laganaro, M., Chetelat-Mabillard, D., & Schnider, A. (2011). Crossover trial of sub-acute computerized aphasia therapy for anomia with the addition of either levodopa or placebo. *Neurorehabilitation and Neural Repair*, *25*, 43–47.

Lester, D. B., Rogers, T. D., & Blaha, C. D. (2010). Acetylcholine-dopamine interactions in the pathophysiology and treatment of CNS disorders. *CNS Neuroscience & Therapeutics*, *16*, 137–162.

Levy, R., & Dubois, B. (2006). Apathy and the functional anatomy of the prefrontal cortex-basal ganglia circuits. *Cerebral Cortex*, *16*, 916–928.

Luria, A. R., & Tsvetkova, L. S. (1968). The mechanism of "dynamic aphasia." *Foundations of Language*, *4*, 296–307.

Mahoney, F. I., & Barthel, D. (1965). Functional evaluation: The Barthel Index. *Maryland State Medical Journal*, *14*, 56–61.

Marin, R. S., Fogel, B. S., Hawkins, J., Duffy, J., & Krupp, B. (1995). Apathy: A treatable syndrome. *Journal of Neuropsychiatry and Clinical Neuroscience*, *7*, 23–30.

Mark, G. P., Shabani, S., Dobbs, L. K., & Hansen, S. T. (2011). Cholinergic modulation of mesolimbic dopamine function and reward. *Physiology and Behavior*, *104*, 76–81.

Mayberg, H. S., Lozano, A. M., Voon, V., McNeely, H. E., Seminowicz, D., Hamani, C., . . . Kennedy, S. H. (2005). Deep brain stimulation for treatment-resistant depression. *Neuron*, *45*, 651–660.

Menke, R., Meinzer, M., Kugel, H., Deppe, M., Baumgartner, A., Schiffbauer, H., . . . Breitenstein, C. (2009). Imaging short and long-term training success in chronic aphasia. *BMC Neuroscience*, *10*, 118.

Paolucci, S. (2008). Epidemiology and treatment of post-stroke depression. *Neuropsychiatric Disease and Treatment*, *4*, 145–154.

Powell, J. H., AlAdawi, S., Morgan, J., & Greenwood, R. J. (1996). Motivational deficits after brain injury: Effects of bromocriptine in 11 patients. *Journal of Neurology Neurosurgery and Psychiatry*, *60*, 416–421.

Ramsberger, G., & Marie, B. (2007). Self-administered cued naming therapy: A single-participant investigation of a computer-based therapy program replicated in four cases. *American Journal of Speech-Language Pathology*, *16*, 343–358.

Raven, J. C. (1976). *Coloured progressive matrices*. San Antonio, TX: Harcourt Assessment.

Raymer, A. M. (2003). Treatment of adynamia in aphasia. *Frontiers in bioscience*, *8*, S845–S851.

Raymer, A. M., Bandy, D., Adair, J. C., Schwartz, R. L., Williamson, D. J. G., Gonzalez Rothi, L. J., . . . Heilman, K. M. (2001). Effects of bromocriptine in a patient with crossed nonfluent aphasia: A case report. *Archives of Physical Medicine and Rehabilitation*, *82*, 139–144.

Reitan, R. M. (1958). Validity of the Trail Making test as an indicator of organic brain damage. *Perceptual Motor Skills*, *8*, 271–276. Also available in: Lezak, M. D., Howieson, D. B., Bigler, E. D. & Tranel, D. (2012). *Neuropsychological assessment* (5th ed.). New York, NY: Oxford University Press.

Robertson, I., Ward, T., Ridgeway, V., & Nimmo-Smith, I. (1994). *The test of everyday attention*. London: Harcourt Assessment.

Robinson, G., Blair, J., & Cipolotti, L. (1998). Dynamic aphasia: An inability to select between competing verbal responses? *Brain*, *121*, 77–89.

Sabe, L., Salvarezza, F., García Cuerva, A., Leiguarda, R., & Starkstein, S. (1995). A randomized, double-blind, placebo-controlled study of bromocriptine in nonfluent aphasia. *Neurology*, *45*, 2272–2274.

Seniów, J., Litwin, M., Litwin, T., Leśniak, M., & Członkowska, A. (2009). New approach to the rehabilitation of post-stroke focal cognitive syndrome: Effect of levodopa combined with speech and language therapy on functional recovery from aphasia. *Journal of the Neurological Sciences, 15*, 214–218.

Starkstein, S. E., & Manes, F. (2000). Apathy and depression following stroke. *CNS Spectrums, 5*, 43–50.

Willems, R. M., & Varley, R. (2010). Neural insights into the relation between language and communication. *Frontiers in Human Neuroscience, 4*. doi:10.3389/fnhum.2010.00203

Whyte, E. M., Lenze, E. J., Butters, M., Skidmore, E., Koenig, K., Dew, M. A., . . . Munin, M. C. (2008). An open-label pilot study of acetylcholinesterase inhibitors to promote functional recovery in elderly cognitively impaired stroke patients. *Cerebrovascular Diseases, 26*, 317–321.

World Health Organisation. (2001). *International Classification of Functioning, Disability and Health* [world wide web] Retrieved February 2013, from http://www.who.int/classifications/icf/en/

APPENDIX A: EXAMPLES OF MCNEMAR CONTINGENCY TABLES: PALPA NAMING

Baseline		✓	x	Total		Baseline		✓	x	Total
30 mg	✓	7	**5**	12	30 mg &	✓	6	**14**	20
No	x	**5**	23	28	S&LT	x	**6**	14	20
S&LT	Total	12	28	40		Total	12	28	40

Baseline		✓	x	Total
End of	✓	9	**22**	31
wash No	x	**3**	6	9
S&LT	Total	12	28	40

Bold lettering indicates numbers of interest for the statistical test.

APPENDIX B: ADDITIONAL ABOVE AND BELOW SCANS TO INDICATE EXTENT OF LESION

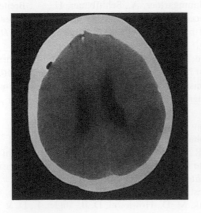
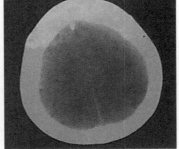

Massed sentence repetition training can augment and speed up recovery of speech production deficits in patients with chronic conduction aphasia receiving donepezil treatment

Marcelo L. Berthier[1], Guadalupe Dávila[1,2], Cristina Green-Heredia[3], Ignacio Moreno Torres[4], Rocío Juárez y Ruiz de Mier[1], Irene De-Torres[1], and Rafael Ruiz-Cruces[1]

[1]Unit of Cognitive Neurology and Aphasia, Centro de Investigaciones Médico-Sanitarias (CIMES), University of Malaga, Malaga, Spain
[2]Area of Psychobiology, Department of Psychology, University of Malaga, Malaga, Spain
[3]Department of Neuroscience, Hospital Quirón, Malaga, Spain
[4]Department of Spanish Language II, University of Malaga, Malaga, Spain

Background: In the past two decades, single-case studies evaluated the effect of massed repetition training to improve speech production and short-term memory deficits in conduction aphasia (CA). Improvements were reported in treated language and memory domains with modest generalisation of gains to spontaneous speech or auditory comprehension. Although these results are encouraging, sentence repetition training has not been compared with distributed speech-language therapy, and no studies have examined the role of pharmacological interventions to enhance gains promoted by these behavioural interventions in CA.

Aims: The effects of massed sentence repetition therapy (MSRT) were compared to those of distributed speech-language therapy (DSLT) in measures of verbal output, short-term memory and repetition in patients with chronic post-stroke CA receiving treatment with the cholinesterase inhibitor donepezil (DP).

Methods and Procedures: Three patients with chronic CA aphasia associated to large left perisylvian infarctions participated in a 28-week open-label study combining DP with DSLT or MSRT. A within-patient design, with baselines across behaviours and a washout period was used. Patients were treated with DP (10 mg/day) combined first with DSLT (16 weeks, 40 hours) and after a washout period (4 weeks) with MSRT (8 weeks, 40 hours). Language functions were assessed with the Western Aphasia Battery and experimental repetition tasks prior to and after DSLT and MSRT.

The authors thank the patients for their cooperation during the study. This study has been supported by a grant from Pfizer and Eisai (Spain) to the corresponding author.

This paper has been presented in part in the Twenty-Sixth Annual International Neuropsychological Society Mid-Year Conference, 16–20 July 2003, Berlin and in the 56th Annual Meeting of the American Academy of Neurology, San Francisco, 24 April–1 May 2004.

Outcomes and Results: Both interventions improved performance in speech production tasks, but better improvements were found with DP-MSRT than with DP-DSLT. Larger treatment effects were found for DP-MSRT in comparison with baselines and DP-DSLT in repetition of word pairs and triplets, and novel and experimental sentences with generalisation of gains to aphasia severity, connected speech and non-treated control sentences.

Conclusions: Combined interventions with DP and two different aphasia therapies (DSLT and MSRT) significantly improved speech production deficits in CA, but DP-MSRT augmented and speeded up most benefits provided by DP-DSLT.

Conduction aphasia (CA) is characterised by a disproportionate deficit in repetition in the context of fluent verbal output and relative sparing of auditory comprehension (Albert, Goodglass, Helm, Rubens, & Alexander, 1981; Berthier, Dávila, García-Casares, & Moreno-Torres, 2014; Kohn, 1992). However, in recent years, CA has been fractionated in a spectrum of syndromes which are to some extent dependent on aphasia severity, moment of aphasia evaluation, type of repetition tasks used, lesion location and availability of compensatory brain mechanisms (Berthier, Lambon Ralph, Pujol, & Green, 2012; Gvion & Friedmann, 2012; Nadeau, 2001). Within this syndromic spectrum, two major types of CA (reproduction and repetition) prevail (Shallice & Warrington, 1977). The reproduction subtype is characterised by phonemic paraphasias in all verbal modalities and recurring production of sequential phonemic approximations to the target word aimed to self-repair errors (*conduite d'approche*), a pattern of deficits variously ascribed to deficits in speech programming (Bernal & Ardila, 2009), output phonological encoding (Kohn, 1992) or combined deficits in sensory-motor integration and phonological short-term memory (Buchsbaum et al., 2011; Hickok, Houde, & Rong, 2011). The repetition subtype is less severe than the previous one because it shows virtually isolated repetition deficits which have been linked to a selective impairment in auditory-verbal short-term memory (AVSTM) (Shallice & Warrington, 1977).

Acute post-stroke CA roughly accounts for 13% of all aphasic syndromes, with most patients achieving good recovery, yet this figure increases (~23%) when chronic aphasic patients are taken into account (Laska, Hellblom, Murray, Kahan, & Von Arbin, 2001) because CA often represents the end-stage of more severe aphasic syndromes (e.g., global aphasia, Wernicke's aphasia) (Kertesz, 1984). In chronic CA, residual phonological errors and self-corrections may hinder verbal output and functional communication, and deficits in AVSTM additionally disrupt comprehension of complex sentences. Moreover, even in patients who attain good outcomes, the profile of CA may latently remain post recovery (Ueno, Saito, Rogers, & Lambon Ralph, 2011), particularly when patients are subjected to demanding testing conditions (Berthier et al., 2012; Jefferies, Crisp, & Lambon Ralph, 2006). Collectively, these findings imply that devising neuroscience-driven interventions for residual CA could be an important area of enquiry. However, despite its prevalence, reports dealing with theoretically motivated treatments for CA are scant. In the next section, we describe interventions aimed to improve speech production and AVSTM in CA.

REPETITION TRAINING IN CONDUCTION APHASIA

In 1833, the Dublin physician Jonathan Osborne (1794–1864) examined repeatedly over the course of a year a young aphasic patient with fluent polyglot jargon, good comprehension of spoken and written words and poor repetition (Breathnach, 2011), a combination of features which Wernicke comprehensively described more than 40 years later under the rubric of CA (De Bleser, Cubelli, & Luzzatti, 1993; Weiller, Bormann, Saur, Musso, & Rijntjes, 2011; Wernicke, 1906, 1977). After the initial evaluation, Osborne recommended his patient "to commence learning to speak like a child repeating first, the letters of the alphabet, and subsequently words, after another person" (Breathnach, 2011, p. 25). In a follow-up evaluation 8 months later, repetition exercises lead to considerable improvements in spontaneous speech and repetition. The beneficial effects of this intervention were overlooked until recently (see below) perhaps because therapies training the most affected language domain (repetition) to improve fluency and content in spontaneous speech were viewed counterproductive. In this context, in a tutorial textbook of acquired aphasia, Taylor Sarno contended "The therapist chooses those techniques or exercises that allow the patient to use preserved skills, thereby increasing the chances for successful performance" (Taylor Sarno, 1998, p. 617). Although Taylor Sarno's recommendation was accepted as a dogma by many speech therapists, recent developments challenge this classical thinking and modern rehabilitation strategies reveal that interventions directed to repair damaged processes are effective (Basso, 2003). For example, Basso suggests that an "Intervention should be targeted to the underlying damaged processes rather than simply treating the presenting symptoms or looking for a strategy that bypasses the deficit" (Basso, 2003, p. 199). Interventions aimed to remediate language deficits in CA have been reported applying traditional techniques (Cubelli, Foresti, & Consolini, 1988; Léger et al., 2002) or modern massed therapies such us Constraint-Induced Aphasia Therapy (CIAT) (Harnish, Neils-Strunjas, Lamy, & Eliassen, 2008; Pulvermüller et al., 2001). Since some interventions in CA tailored to improve speech production also trained other language domains (reading aloud, picture naming) besides repetition (Cubelli et al., 1988; Léger et al., 2002), these studies are not reviewed here.

In the past two decades, several single-case studies used repetition exercises to improve speech production and AVSTM in CA. Kohn, Smith and Arsenaut (1990) were the first researchers that used sentence repetition exercises in a patient with a moderately severe chronic reproduction CA who had greater speech fluency in repetition than in conversation. The authors selected repetition as the training strategy because they wanted to increase speech fluency rather than accuracy in word production. Two sets of 20 sentences were constructed. One set included sentences rich in semantic content and was composed of substantives and verbs (e.g., "She was there"), whereas the other set was composed of sentences containing pronouns, adverbs and functor verbs (e.g., "Tom played ball"). After two months of sentence repetition exercises carried out at home with the help of family members, improvements were documented in sentence repetition with generalisation of benefits to picture description. The authors concluded that benefits provided by repetition exercises resulted from improvement in phonemic planning in all output modalities rather than from gains in AVSTM (Kohn et al., 1990).

Francis, Clark, and Humphreys (2003) trained word and sentence repetition to improve sentence comprehension in a patient with mild receptive aphasia associated to recurrent strokes. Gains after treatment were observed in digit span, long-term word recognition memory, sentence repetition and Token Test. However, since the patient had suffered recurrent stroke episodes, it has been argued that spontaneous improvement may have played a role in the recovery process (Salis, 2012).

Majerus, Van der Kaa, Renard, Van der Linden, and Poncelet (2005) treated a patient with a phonological short-term memory disorder in two phases. In the initial phase, the patient was asked to repeat pairs of bi-syllabic words or non-words immediately after hearing the stimuli. When the patient achieved a stabilisation in phonological production, delayed repetition tasks (repetition after a 5-second filled interval) that required holding meaningful and meaningless phonological information in AVSTM were used. The patient was treated during 16 months (twice per week) and modest improvements were found in digit and non-word span, non-word repetition and rhyme judgements. Also, the patient had the personal impression of better comprehension in conversational contexts involving more than two partners.

Koenig-Bruhin and Studer-Eichenberger (2007) treated a stroke patient with chronic repetition CA. The purpose was to examine whether deficits of the temporary storage of verbal information could be improved with sentence repetition exercises. Therefore, they trained repetition of sentences that were of four to seven words long with increasing delays between the stimulus and response. The control task consisted of repeating words of four to six words without delay. Treatment significantly improved sentence repetition, and gains were generalised to sentence length in oral production and spans for digits and bi-syllabic words. These findings were interpreted in the frame of the interactive spreading activation model of speech processing as reflecting a slowing down in activation decay (Koening-Bruhin & Studer-Eichenberger, 2007).

In a comprehensive study, Kalinyak-Fliszar, Kohen, and Martin (2011) trained repetition to improve AVSTM and executive processing in a patient with chronic CA using a multiple-baseline, multiple-probe design across behaviours. These researchers used repetition of words and non-words in immediate and delayed conditions. Gains in repetition performance were mostly restricted to treated items, but post-treatment measures of language ability indicated improvements in single and multiple word-processing tasks, verbal working memory tasks and verbal span. Taken together, these results suggest that treating these deficits directly with repetition training may improve speech production (repetition), AVSTM and executive-attentional processes, presumably by reinforcing activation and maintenance of linguistic information in AVSTM (Kalinyak-Fliszar et al., 2011; Koening-Bruhin & Studer-Eichenberger, 2007).

WHY TRAINING REPETITION IN CONDUCTION APHASIA HELPS?

The abovementioned strategy of training repetition to improve speech production and AVSTM deficits is based on scientific knowledge gathered from lesion studies (Gold & Kertesz, 2001; Kohn et al., 1990; Martin, Saffran, & Dell, 1994; Schlaug, Marchina, & Norton, 2009; Zipse, Norton, Marchina, & Schlaug, 2012) and computational network modelling (Dell, Martin, & Schwartz, 2007). Collectively, results from these studies suggest that the functional mechanisms suitable of reparation in CA are a variable combination of pathological reduction of network connection strength, rapid decay of activation in semantic-lexical-phonological networks and restricted AVSTM (Gold & Kertesz, 2001; Jefferies, Sage, & Ralph, 2007; Kalinyak-

Fliszar et al., 2011; Koening-Bruhin & Studer-Eichenberger, 2007; Martin, 1996; Martin & Saffran, 2002). Failure of these mechanisms can be inferred even in patients with mild CA who, in spite of being able to repeat single words with ease (Caplan & Waters, 1992), show abnormal repetition performance when task demands are increased (repetition of word lists and sentences, delayed repetition) (Jefferies et al., 2007). It has been contended that auditory repetition under stressing conditions may adversely impact performance because connection strength and maintenance of language traces in dysfunctional areas of the left hemisphere are unstable (Martin et al., 1994; Martin & Saffran, 2002) with little room for natural compensation by contralateral homotopic regions (see data from patient JVA in Berthier et al., 2012). In support, knowledge from both computational network modelling (Ueno et al. 2011) and resting state functional magnetic resonance imaging (rs$f$MRI) in patients with focal brain lesions to critical areas (e.g., connectors) (Gratton, Nomura, Pérez, & D'Esposito, 2012) shows that disruption of network architecture impacts in nearby and remote components of the networks and even in contralesional areas. In chronic CA patients with extensive left hemisphere lesions, these remote effects may result in reduced function and failure to successfully recruit alternative neural systems (e.g., right perisylvian white matter pathways). Therefore, implementing massed and highly focused therapies, like sentence repetition training, might be useful to facilitate the use of alternatives routes when the original ones are enduringly damaged. Massed sentence repetition therapy aims, as other neuroscience-inspired therapies (CIAT) (Pulvermüller et al., 2001), the potentiation of both associationist (or coincident) Hebbian learning (Hebb, 1949) and interconnectivity of language with other processes (attention, executive function, motor system) as well as the attenuation of the deleterious effect of learned non-use in the persistence of cognitive deficits after brain injury (see Pulvermüller & Berthier, 2008).

The neural mechanisms promoting recovery from speech production deficits in response to sentence repetition/imitation training have been examined in patients with non-fluent Broca's aphasia and improvements were related to recruitment of left ventral stream (inferior fronto-occipital fasciculus [IFOF]) when this white matter bundle was spared by the lesion (Fridriksson et al., 2012) or right hemisphere networks in cases with large left hemisphere lesions (Schlaug et al., 2009; Zipse et al., 2012). A complimentary participation of the mirror neuron system (Ertelt & Binkofski, 2012; Small, Buccino, & Solodkin, 2010) or visual areas (Fridriksson et al., 2012) has been suggested as well. However, at present, the biological roots of recovery from CA have not been investigated, yet the beneficial role of repetition training can be tentatively inferred from the abovementioned data (cf. Zipse et al., 2012). Before addressing this topic, we will briefly outline the current state-of-the-art of the neural mechanisms underpinning normal language repetition and maintenance of the verbal trace in short-term memory. This would allow the elaboration of a conceptual framework for understanding the neural mechanisms instantiating residual repetition in CA and the development of rehabilitation strategies for exploiting this residual capacity to facilitate recovery.

The role of cortical areas (inferior parietal lobule, superior temporal gyrus) and white matter pathways (arcuate fasciculus [AF], IFOF) underpinning repetition is still a matter of controversy (Bernal & Ardila, 2009; Berthier et al., 2012; Dick & Tremblay, 2012; Saur et al., 2008). Some authors defend the role of cortical areas (e.g., Bernal & Ardila, 2009), whereas others maintain that perisylvian white matter tracts (AF, IFOF) are the anatomic signatures of repetition (Berthier et al., 2012;

Friederici & Gierhan, 2013; Geschwind, 1965; Gierhan, 2013; Rijntjes, Weiller, Bormann, & Musso, 2012; Saur et al., 2008). Diffusion tensor imaging (DTI) studies have examined the anatomy and connectivity of white matter tracts subserving repetition (Catani, Jones, & Ffytche, 2005; Catani & Thiebaut de Schotten, 2012; Catani et al., 2007; Saur et al., 2008). DTI studies not only allow delineation of the fine architecture of long-distance and short-distance white matter tracts (for review see Geva, Correia, & Warburton, 2011), but can also reveal anatomic asymmetries which might be related to differences in repetition performance in normal and brain-damaged subjects (Berthier et al., in press; Catani et al., 2007). Long-distance white matter tracts binding remote cortical language sites are segregated in a dual stream architecture (dorsal and ventral streams), wherein the role of the dorsal auditory stream system (AF, superior longitudinal fasciculus) is to monitor auditory-motor integration of speech by allowing a fast and automated preparation of copies of the perceived speech input (Peschke, Ziegler, Kappes, & Baumgaertner, 2009; Rijntjes et al., 2012; Saur et al., 2008). The ventral auditory stream (IFOF, extreme capsulae and uncinate fasciculus) participates in the mapping of sounds onto meaning (Cloutman, 2012; Peschke et al., 2009; Saur et al., 2008) although the precise functional role of every tract is still controversial (Duffau, Gatignol, Moritz-Gasser, & Mandonnet, 2009; Harvey, Wei, Ellmore, Hamilton, & Schnur, 2013). Word and sentence information temporarily activated in the dorsal and ventral language processing networks is presumably controlled and maintained via a left fronto-parietal attention processing network (Majerus, 2013; Majerus et al., 2012).

Anatomically, the dorsal stream (AF) is more lateralised to the left hemisphere than other white matter tracts including the ventral stream (IFOF) (Hickok & Poeppel, 2007; Nucifora, Verma, Melhem, Gur, & Gur, 2005) and the former also has individual differences in its intra- and inter-hemispheric architecture (Catani & Thiebaut de Schotten, 2012; Catani et al., 2007). The most common anatomical pattern of the AF is characterised by extreme leftward lateralisation of the direct segment and lack of this segment in the right hemisphere, a configuration that predominates in males. A second pattern has been identified having a less strongly lateralised long direct segment in the left hemisphere than the previous pattern and it is associated with a vestigial right hemisphere direct component. The third pattern, usually documented in females, has a roughly symmetrical distribution of direct segments (Catani & Mesulam, 2008). Data from healthy subjects revealed that the auditory-motor integration needed to learn new words depends on the activity of the left AF (López-Barroso et al., 2013) and also that superior verbal learning through repetition correlates with the symmetrical pattern (Catani et al., 2007). The advantage for certain cognitive functions (verbal learning) amongst individuals having symmetrical AF raises the possibility that left brain-damaged patients praised with a well-developed direct segment of the right AF may be ideal candidates to rehabilitation strategies tailored to exploit repetition through this pathway (Schlaug et al., 2009; Zipse et al., 2012). In this context, DTI performed before and after Melodic Intonation Therapy (Sparks, Helm, & Albert, 1974)[1] and CIAT (Pulvermüller &

---

[1] Melodic Intonation Therapy (MIT) is a rehabilitation technique commonly used to treat patients with non-fluent speech production and preserved comprehension (Broca's aphasia) resulting from left hemisphere damage (Sparks et al., 1974). MIT engages relatively preserved functions (melody, rhythm and formulaic language) dependent upon right perisylvian white matter tracts and corticostriatal activity to improve verbal output and communication (Schlaug et al., 2009; Stahl, Henseler, Turner, Geyer, & Kotz, 2013; Zipse et al., 2012)

Berthier, 2008; Pulvermüller et al., 2001) in patients with Broca's aphasia showed that post-therapy gains in language performance correlated with structural plasticity of the right AF (Breier, Juranek, & Papanicolaou, 2011; Schlaug et al., 2009; Zipse et al., 2012).

Verbal repetition entails the imitation of not only incoming auditory stimuli, but also visual signals through action observation (Iacoboni et al., 1999; Keysers et al., 2003; Kohler et al., 2002). Imitation, action understanding, learning and language may depend partially on the activity of the mirror neuron system. The mirror neurons are located in Brodmann's area 44, superior temporal gyrus and inferior parietal lobule. Since these cortical areas are interconnected through the auditory dorsal stream (AF), it has been contended that the mirror neuron system and the dorsal white matter bundle are tightly intertwined (Arbib, 2010; Corballis, 2010). This would imply that interventions combining repetition of auditory signals with visual stimuli (viewing the mouth of a person speaking aloud the to-be-repeated material) would create a more compelling scenario for rehabilitation than repeating auditory stimuli alone. Fridriksson and colleagues (Fridriksson et al., 2012) found that audio-visual feedback improved more spontaneous speech than audio-only feedback in patients with chronic Broca's aphasia. A similar line of thought has been exploited to devise a new intervention (IMITATE) to train repetition and imitation of audio-visual stimuli in aphasic patients (Lee, Fowler, Rodney, Cherney, & Small, 2010; Small et al., 2010). Up to now, IMITATE has not been used to treat CA patients, but based on the abovementioned role of repetition training in previous cases, it is tempting to envision that this technique would also apply for CA patients. Despite the improvements provided by auditory repetition training in spontaneous speech (Kohn et al., 1990), sentence comprehension (Francis et al., 2003) and AVSTM (Kalinyak-Fliszar et al., 2011), it can be wondered whether complementary interventions in CA may enhance recovery further. One potential strategy, which is discussed below, is strengthening language gains provided by aphasia therapy with pharmacotherapy.

CAN CHOLINERGIC MODULATION BOOSTS APHASIA THERAPY EFFECTS IN CONDUCTION APHASIA?

The efficacy of aphasia therapy is well proven (Basso, 2003; Cherney, 2012; Varley, 2011). Nonetheless, developing complementary strategies to augment and speed up its benefits is advantageous (Allen, Mehta, McClure, & Teasell, 2012; Berthier & Pulvermüller, 2011; Small & Llano, 2009). Amongst these strategies, drug therapy is emerging as a promissory option to augment cognitive function in both healthy individuals (Husain & Mehta, 2011) and brain-damaged patients (Berthier, Pulvermüller, Dávila, Casares, & Gutiérrez, 2011; Shisler, Baylis, & Frank, 2000; Small & Llano, 2009). The basic idea behind using drugs to treat aphasia is that focal brain lesions interrupt the ascending projections of major neurotransmitter systems (e.g., acetylcholine, dopamine) from basal forebrain or brainstem to cerebral cortex and subcortical nuclei causing synaptic depression in both perilesional areas and remote regions (Berthier & Pulvermüller, 2011; Gotts & Plaut, 2002). Thus, drugs enhancing or leveraging the activity of neurotransmitters in dysfunctional but still viable speech and language areas can improve aphasic deficits. Moreover, since executive functions and attention resources may be abnormal in patients with CA (Kalinyak-Fliszar et al., 2011), restoring neurotransmitter activity in non-eloquent areas mediating these functions with drugs (DP) that modulate these cognitive functions (Sarter, Bruno, & Givens, 2003; Sarter, Hasselmo, Bruno, & Givens, 2005) may contribute to augment the gains obtained with repetition therapy. In the same vein, improving cholinergic activity in other non-language regions (e.g., cingulate gyrus, orbitofrontal cortex, basal ganglia) can likewise contribute to indirectly boost language functions by improving functional communication, cognitive control, goal-directed behaviour and mood (Berthier, 2012; Whyte et al., 2008).

Cholinergic agents are commonly used to treat Alzheimer's disease (Birks, 2006). On the basis of their beneficial effects on language deficits and repetitive verbalisation (statements, stories) in patients with Alzheimer's disease (Asp et al., 2006; Rockwood, Fay, Jarrett, & Asp, 2007) and cognitive deficits of vascular origin (Barrett et al., 2011), the use of cholinergic drugs (donepezil and galantamine) have been extended to treat post-stroke aphasia. Drugs targeting the cholinergic system were used for the first time to treat aphasic deficits in the late 1960s (Luria, Naydyn, Tsvetkova, & Vinarskaya, 1969), and these agents recently led to evidence for beneficial effects on naming and other language functions in post-stroke aphasia (Berthier et al., 2006; Berthier, Hinojosa, Martín, & Fernández, 2003; Chen et al., 2010; Hong, Shin, Lim, Lee, & Huh, 2012; Tanaka, Albert, Fujita, Nonaka, & Yokoyama, 2006). Anatomical studies in the human brain reveal that the perisylvian language cortex is innervated by cholinergic fibres emanating from the nucleus basalis of Meynert or *Ch4* group (Boban, Kostovic, & Simic, 2006; Mesulam, 2004; Simić et al., 1999) and also that cholinergic activity is greater in the left temporal lobe than in the right one (Klein & Albert, 2004). Basal forebrain cholinergic projections are not only directed to the cortical language core as they also innervate more discrete cortical fields (e.g., cingulate gyrus, precuneus, orbitofrontal cortex) and cholinergic projections arising from the upper brainstem modulate the activity of thalamus and basal ganglia (Mesulam, Mash, Hersh, Bothwell, & Geula, 1992).

The modulation of the cholinergic system in post-stroke aphasia seems to be beneficial even when unpaired with aphasia therapy (Chen et al., 2010; Hong et al., 2012). Nevertheless, in light of the growing experimental data showing that cortical map plasticity induced by cholinergic agents can be enhanced further as soon as the cholinergic stimulation is administered in combination with behavioural training (Ramanathan, Tuszynski, & Conner, 2009), recent intervention trials in aphasia successfully combined cholinergic stimulation with aphasia therapy (Berthier et al., 2003, 2006). The mechanisms by which cholinergic stimulation promote recovery from aphasia are still unknown, but several mechanisms has been proposed to explain how cholinergic modulation facilitates access to target words during behavioural training including reversion of synaptic depression (Gotts & Plaut, 2002), reduction of spreading activation of competitors (Foster et al., 2012) and increase of speed and accuracy of information processing (Berthier & Green, 2007). In other words, it is possible that cholinergic modulation makes brain structure a more fertile ground for behavioural intervention.

THE PRESENT STUDY

The duration and intensity with which aphasia therapy need to be administered is an important area of ongoing research, yet to date few studies have addressed the impact of distributed as compared to massed aphasia therapies on outcomes and available results are controversial (see Cherney, Patterson, & Raymer, 2011;

Harnish et al., 2008; Martins et al., 2013; Sage, Snell, & Lambon Ralph, 2011). There is general agreement that aphasia therapy in stroke patients is beneficial when evidence-based protocols of intervention are used (Basso & Macis, 2011; Bhogal, Teasell, & Speechley, 2003; Cappa et al., 2005; Cicerone et al., 2011; Robey, 1998). However, some limitations not related to the essential characteristics of the interventions still exist. To name a few, aphasia therapy is time consuming and expensive (Berthier, 2005), and these difficulties would explain, amongst other reasons, the gap that exists between what the research on aphasia therapy recommends as the appropriate amount of treatment and the actual provision in several countries (Code & Petheram, 2011). Moreover, adherence to prolonged aphasia therapy is not always feasible due to logistic problems (e.g., transportation difficulties). Finally, unwillingness to participate and abandonment of therapy are commonly reported in elderly patients (Basso & Macis, 2011). Therefore, the idea that the benefits provided by aphasia therapy can be augmented and speeded up using emerging approaches (e.g., drugs, transcranial and electrical brain stimulation) needs to be explored. For example, distributed speech-language therapy (DSLT) is not particularly useful in chronic aphasia, but potentiating its beneficial effects with drugs has been associated with better outcomes (Berthier et al., 2003, 2006). Following the same line of thought, the next step is to know if the same amount of therapy but administered in a shorter period of time combining massed, theoretically motivated interventions with drugs may yield better outcomes. Interestingly enough, preliminary evidence from a single patient with chronic CA demonstrated greater gains with massed therapy than with distributed therapy, and benefits provided by the former intervention correlated with increased left basal ganglia and right hemisphere recruitment (Harnish et al., 2008). Therefore, to gain further knowledge on the integration of emerging therapies with classical interventions, this study compares the efficacy of two different behavioural interventions (distributed and massed aphasia therapies) in three patients with chronic CA receiving drug treatment with the cholinergic enhancer donepezil (DP).[2]

METHOD

Participants

The three male patients who participated in the present study had been included in a 20-week open-label pilot trial evaluating the effects of DP and DSLT in chronic post-stroke aphasia (total sample = 11 patients) (Berthier et al., 2003). Eligible participants for that trial had to meet the following criteria: (1) native speaker of Spanish, (2) right handed, (3) between the ages of 18 and 70 years, (4) chronic aphasia (> 1 year) and (5) left hemisphere stroke lesion. After the last end point of the trial (washout phase, week 20), these three patients were invited to take part in an extension phase (8 weeks) combining DP with MSRT. All three patients were

---

[2] Donepezil is a centrally acting reversible acetylcholinesterase inhibitor. It inhibits the enzyme (acetylcholinesterase) that breaks down acetylcholine in the synaptic cleft, thus increasing both the level and duration of action of endogenous acetylcholine. Although donepezil is only authorised for the treatment of Alzheimer's disease, it has been tested (off label use) in other cognitive disorders, including vascular dementia and vascular and degenerative aphasias. Donepezil is safe and well-tolerated in patients with these disorders. Nonetheless, it should be used with caution in patients with cardiac conduction disturbances, chronic obstructive pulmonary disease, severe bronchial asthma, severe cardiac arrhythmias and sick sinus syndrome.

selected because they had relatively homogeneous language deficits of lesser severity (baseline WAB-AQ score: [mean ± SD] 72.4 ± 9.6) than the other eight patients (baseline WAB-AQ score: [mean ± SD] 45.3 ± 13.4) (Berthier, 2005) and because they had relatively homogeneous lesion locations on MRI scans.

Case descriptions

Patient RRM. This patient was a 51-year-old right-handed male, who left school at 15 and had previously been a newspaper worker. He suffered a large left fronto-temporo-parietal infarction 17 months before trial enrolment. In the acute post-stroke period, he had a right hemiparesis and global aphasia which gradually evolved to a severe CA with mild apraxia of speech. Aphasia therapy during one year (two sessions a week) partially improved auditory comprehension and non-fluent speech production. On baseline evaluation with the Western Aphasia Battery (WAB) (Kertesz, 1982), his language deficits were consistent with CA. RRM's speech was dysfluent and contaminated by word retrieval problems, neologisms, phonological and formal errors (Table 1). Further testing with selected subtests of the Psycholinguistic Assessments of Language Processing in Aphasia (PALPA) (Kay, Lesser, & Coltheart, 1992; Valle & Cuetos, 1995) disclosed a relative preservation of auditory comprehension (words, lexical decisions and sentences) but input phonology (auditory minimal word and non-word pairs) was abnormal. Picture naming was moderately impaired. Word repetition, though impaired, was less affected than non-word and digit repetition. Sentence repetition was moderately impaired.

TABLE 1
Background language testing

Test	RRM	VRG	JTO
Western aphasia battery			
Aphasia quotient (range: 0–100)	61.6	76	79.8
Information content (max: 10)	7	8	9
Fluency (max: 10)	5[a]	6	8
Comprehension (max: 10)	9.7	9.3	9.1
Repetition (max: 10)	4.6	4.2	6
Naming (max: 10)	4.5	8.5	7.8
PALPA			
Non-word minimal pairs ($n = 56$)	46 (.82)	47 (.84)	41 (.73)
Word minimal pairs ($n = 56$)	48 (.86)	48 (.86)	46 (.82)
Auditory lexical decision ($n = 160$)	154 (.96)	150 (.94)	148 (.92)
Repetition, syllable length ($n = 24$)	17*	21**	20***
Repetition: non-words ($n = 24$)	7	9	10
Spoken word–picture matching ($n = 40$)	40 (1.0)	40 (1.0)	38 (.95)
Sentence comprehension ($n = 60$)	55 (.92)	49 (.87)	48 (.80)
Naming by frequency ($n = 60$)	30 (.50)	54 (.90)	45 (.75)
Digit production	2	3	2

Patients are arranged in order of Aphasia Quotient scores derived from four subtests (spontaneous speech, comprehension, repetition, and naming). The combination of fluent speech production (WAB fluency score ≥ 5), relatively preserved comprehension (WAB comprehension score > 7) and impaired repetition (WAB repetition score < 6.9) indicates conduction aphasia.
[a]This patient additionally had mild apraxia of speech (Ardila & Roselli, 1990) and his verbal production was less fluent than usually reported (Broca-like CA) (Song et al., 2011). Word repetition versus non-word repetition: *$p = .01$; **$p = .001$; ***$p = .008$ (Fisher Exact Test, two-tailed).

Patient VRG. This patient was a 52-year-old right-handed male, who left school at 16 and had previously worked as an administrative. He suffered a large left fronto-tem-poro-parietal infarction 22 months before referral for the present trial. In the acute period, he had a right hemiparesis and global aphasia. He gradually recovered with speech-language therapy and physiotherapy, but on referral to our unit, he had a dystonic right hand and foot posture and a moderate CA (Table 1). On the WAB, his speech was fluent and free of phonological paraphasias but showed word retrieval problems and occasional formal errors. Further testing with PALPA subtests disclosed a relative preservation of auditory comprehension (lexical decisions and words) except for discriminating minimal word and non-word pairs and sentence comprehension. Picture naming was preserved. Word repetition was mildly impaired but much better than non-word and digit repetition. Sentence repetition was moderately impaired.

Patient JTO. This patient was a 72-year-old right-handed male who suffered a left fronto-temporo-parietal infarction 13 months before referral for participating in this drug trial. He had worked as an attorney until his retirement at age 65. In the acute post-stroke phase, he showed a rapidly resolving right hemiparesis and a global aphasia. Aphasia therapy (two sessions a week) was beneficial but gains reached a plateau after 6 months of treatment. On baseline evaluation, he had a moderate CA (see Table 1). On picture description from the WAB, his speech was fluent and free of phonological paraphasias. However, his utterances were punctuated by word retrieval problems, formal, perseverative and semantic errors. On PALPA subtests, he had a relative preservation of auditory comprehension (lexical decisions and words), except for dis-criminating minimal word and non-word pairs and sentence comprehension. Picture naming was moderately impaired. Word repetition was mildly impaired but much better than non-word and digit repetition. Sentence repetition was impaired.

Neuroimaging. MRIs at the chronic stage were performed in all three patients on different 1.5-T scanners. Areas of infarctions were manually drawn on representative axial slices (templates 3, 12, 18, 26) from the MRIcron software (www.mccausland-center.sc.edu/mricro/mricron) (Rorden, 2005). Lesion mapping was done by a radi-ologist (RR-C) who was blind to patients' demographic and clinical information using a modification of the methodology described by Gardner et al. (Gardner et al., 2012). Lesion size was estimated by overlying a standardised grid of squares (square area .1225 cm) onto each patient's template of the left hemisphere (grid area: 10.29 cm) and working out the percentage of squares damaged relative to undamaged parts of the left hemisphere (Gardner et al., 2012). Total or partial involvement of cortical and subcortical regions was registered (Table 2), and Brodmann's areas involved by the lesions were identified in every patient with the aid of the Brain Voyager Brain Tutor (www.brainvoyager.com/BrainTutor.html). Regions of ischaemic gliosis sur-rounding the infarctions were also drawn on the basis of increased signal in T_2-weighted images. The relative involvement of perisylvian white matter tracts (AF and IFOF) was estimated using an atlas of human brain connections (Catani & Thiebaut de Schotten, 2012).

Large parts of the left middle and superior temporal gyri, supramarginal gyrus, dorsal insula and white matter corresponding to the dorsal stream (AF) were severely damaged in all patients. The ventral insula (posterior and middle parts) through which the ventral stream (IFOF) runs was severely damaged in two patients (RRM and JTO) and mildly affected in the remaining patient. Patient RRM had the more

TABLE 2
Lesion analysis

Patient	% of damage[a]	STG BA 22	BA 41	BA 42	MTG BA 21	ITG BA 20	AG BA 39	SMG BA 40	POT BA 37	DLPFC BA 9/46	orbIFG BA 47	trIFG BA 45	opIFG BA 44	Ventral insula	Dorsal insula	Dorsal stream	Ventral stream	Basal ganglia
RRM	27	2	2	2	2	–	1	2	–	–	–	–	1	1	2	2	2	1
VRG	14.3	2	2	2	2	–	–	2	–	–	–	–	1	–	2	2	1	1
JTO	14.1	2	2	2	2	–	–	2	–	–	–	–	–	2	2	2	2	1

Quantification of lesion location: 2 = complete involvement/serious damage to cortical/subcortical region; 1 = partial involvement/mild damage to cortical/subcortical region.

Abbreviations of cortical regions: STG = superior temporal gyrus; ITG = inferior temporal gyrus; AG = angular gyrus; SMG = supramarginal gyrus; POT = posterior occipito-temporal area; DLPFC = dorsolateral prefrontal cortex; orbIFG = pars orbitalis of the inferior frontal gyrus; trIFG = pars triangularis of the inferior frontal gyrus; opIFG = pars opercularis of the inferior frontal gyrus.

[a]Lesion size was estimated by overlying a standardised grid of squares onto each patient's template and working out the percentage of squares damaged relative to undamaged parts of the left hemisphere (Gardner et al., 2012).

severe aphasia and the largest area of damage due to a frontal extension of the infarct, whereas less severe aphasia and relatively smaller lesions were documented in patients VRG and JTO. Further details of the patients' lesions are shown in Table 2 and Figure 1.

Study design

As already stated, language data from these three patients were initially included in a group analysis together with data from the other eight patients (total sample = 11) (Berthier et al., 2003). For the present case-series study, data from the initial phase (weeks 0 to 16), washout (weeks 16 to 20) and extension phase (weeks 20 to 28) were analysed in an individual basis, except for treatment effects which were analysed as a group using Cohen's d statistics (Cohen, 1988). Therefore, a within-patient design, with baselines across behaviours and a washout period was adopted (Gast & Ledford, 2009). An A_1-BC-A_2-BD was used wherein A_1 represented the initial baseline testing, BC was the combination of DP with DSLT, A_2 was a new baseline after the washout period and BD was the combination of DP with MSRT. Multiple baseline evaluations before initiating the trial were not performed because language deficits in all patients were considered stable by virtue of their long aphasia duration (>1 year) and because they had reached a plateau with previous interventions which motivated referral for participation in the trial. The analysis of an A_1-BC-A_2-BD design led to three treatment comparisons, and three effect sizes were computed to represent the three demonstrations of experimental effect. These effect sizes relate to the phase comparisons of A_1-BC (baseline to the first intervention phase—week 0 vs. week 16), BC-A_2 (the first treatment phase to the washout, second baseline—week 16 vs. week 20), and A_2-BD (the second baseline to the second intervention phase—week 20 vs. week 28). Further comparisons between A_1 and BD and BC and BD were performed. Language evaluations were performed at baselines A_1 (week 0) and A_2 (week 20) and at end points BC (week 16) and BD (week 28). The study was performed according to the Declaration of Helsinki and the protocol was approved by the Local Community Ethics Committee for Clinical Trials. This study was conducted as an independent research project funded by Pfizer/Eisai, Spain, and it was designed, conducted and controlled by the principal investigator (MLB).

Drug treatment

In both drug phases of the study, all patients received DP (5 mg once a day) during a 4-week titration phase followed by a 12-week maintenance phase (week 4 to week 16) (BC) and by a 4-week maintenance phase (week 24 to week 28) (BD). Drug treatment and aphasia therapy were interrupted during the washout period (week 20 to week 24). Compliance was determined at every visit by tablet counts. DP tablets were provided by Pfizer/Eisai, Spain. The detection of potential adverse events was monitored during the trial.

Aphasia therapies

Distributed speech-language therapy (DSLT). All three patients received DSLT at the same rehabilitation centre and were treated by the same speech therapist. DSLT followed a syndrome-specific standard approach and the therapeutic repertoire

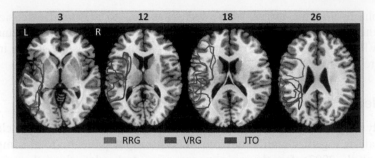

Figure 1. Representative axial slices (3, 12, 18, 26) from the MRIcron software (www.mccauslandcenter.sc. edu/mricro/mricron) (Rorden, 2005) depicting the full extension of lesions in each patient. See further details in text and lesion topography in Table 2. [To view this figure in colour, please see the online version of this Journal].

ranged from exercises involving naming, repetition, sentence completion, following commands, spoken object-picture matching and conversations on topics of the patients' own choice (Basso, 2003; Basso, Forbes, & Boller, 2013; Pulvermüller et al., 2001). In this trial phase, patients received DP-DSLT during 16 weeks and the total hours of therapy was 40 (~2.30 h/wk).

Massed sentence repetition therapy (MSRT). MSRT consisted of sentence repetition exercises and these were practiced at home where the patients were required to repeat audio-taped sentences. Patients received explanations on how to perform MSRT and one training practice session by a speech therapist. There were two sets of 20 sentences similar to the ones used by Kohn et al. (1990). One set was composed of sentences rich in semantic content (substantives, verbs) (e.g., "The boy runs"), whereas the other set included sentences mainly composed of pronouns, verbs and functor verbs (e.g., "She thinks about everything"). Sentence length in both sets ranged from 2 to 7 words. In this phase, patients received DP-MSRT during 8 weeks and the total number hours of therapy was 40 (~ 1 h/day, 5 days a week).

Control sentences. To evaluate possible generalisation of gains provided by MSRT, patients were asked to repeat a control list of 60 sentences which were not included in the therapy sets. Sentences length also ranged from 2 to 7 words (e.g., "give me bread"; "the girl sleeps in the sofa"). Testing was conducted only at baseline A_2 (week 20) and end point BD (week 28).

Outcome measures

Aphasia severity: Western aphasia battery-aphasia quotient. To rate changes in the severity of aphasia the WAB-AQ was used. The WAB-AQ is a measure of aphasia severity which has been shown sensible enough to detect longitudinal changes in previous drug trials with different cholinesterase inhibitors (Berthier et al., 2003, 2006; Chen et al., 2010; Hong et al., 2012). Reductions in the WAB-AQ scores ≥ 5 at end points (BC and BD) in comparison to baselines (A_1 and A_2) were considered a positive response to the intervention (Berthier et al., 2011; Cherney, Erickson, & Small, 2010).

Connected speech production. To examine connected speech production, speech samples in baselines and post-treatment phases were obtained from the picture description (picnic scene) of the WAB during a time limit of 5 minutes. All descriptions were audio-taped and transcribed. Since measures to rating spontaneous speech (fluency and information content) of the WAB are to a certain extent unreliable, speech samples were analysed for percentage of correct information units (%CIU) defined as non-redundant content words that convey correct information about the stimulus (Marchina et al., 2011; Nicholas & Brookshire, 1993; Zipse et al., 2012) using the following formula: number of CIUs/number of words × 100. According to Nicholas and Brookshire (1993) to be classified as CIUs, words should not only be intelligible in context, but also be accurate, relevant and informative with respect to the stimulus. Meaningless utterances, perseverations, paraphasias and other inappropriate information (exclamations) were counted as words, but not classified as CIUs.

Repetition tasks

Word and non-word repetition. Two subtests of PALPA were used. Repetition of words was assessed with the Repetition: Syllable Length (test 7), and non-words with the Repetition: Non-words (test 8).

Word pair repetition. To assess the effect on performance during word repetition when the memory load is increased, patients were required to repeat word pairs in three different conditions: (1) no delay direct (e.g., "house-flower") (*n* = 55), (2) no delay inverted (e.g., "flower-house") (*n* = 55), and (3) unfilled delay (after a delay of 5 seconds unfilled by the neither the patient or researcher) (*n* = 55) (Gold & Kertesz, 2001; Martin, Saffran, & Dell, 1996).

Word triplet repetition. To assess the influence of interventions on lexical-semantic information when the demand of the AVSTM is increased, all patients were asked to repeat word triplets. This task is a modification of the one used by McCarthy and Warrington (1987) in patients with CA. The present repetition battery included three lists of high-frequency words and three lists of low-frequency words (Berthier, 2001). Two sets of 60 three-word lists (verb-adjective-noun) were constructed. These were composed of word strings of increasing semantic richness that is from non-organised to organised semantic information. Two 20 three-word lists (List 1: 60 high-frequency words; List 4: 60 low-frequency words) consisted of random word combinations (e.g., "walk-shiny-pools"). Two other 20 three-words lists (List 2: 60 high-frequency words; List 5: 60 low-frequency words) conveyed loosely constrained meaningful information (e.g., "crawl-slow-baby"), and two other 20 three-word lists (List 3: 60 high-frequency words; List 6: 60 low-frequency words) conveyed closely constrained meaningful information (e.g., "eat-green-apple"). Words were read at a rate of one per second, and patients were required to repeat the words in the order given by the examiner. Responses were scored for the number of lists repeated verbatim in each condition and for the number of words repeated accurately as a function of serial position (initial, medial and final) in the list, irrespective of whether the list was repeated accurately or not.

Repetition of clichés and novel sentences. Patients with CA tend to show better performance on repeating novel sentences than idiomatic clichés, because they can access meaning during repetition of the former type of sentences (McCarthy & Warrington, 1984). To explore this dissociation, all three patients were asked to repeat familiar idiomatic phrases of Spanish (*n* = 40) taken from the 150 Famous

Clichés of Spanish Language (Junceda, 1981) and a set of novel, control phrases ($n = 40$) that were constructed following the methodology described by Cum and Ellis (1999). Novel phrases were derived from the idiomatic phrases by replacing one to three content words in each phrase by other words matched in length of words and word frequency. Both sets of phrases (clichés and novel) were randomised and read aloud to patients one at a time.

RESULTS

Aphasia severity: Western aphasia battery-aphasia quotient

Individual analyses showed that the aphasia severity measured with the WAB-AQ improved significantly in comparison with baseline assessment (A_1) with both interventions in all patients (DP-DSLT: RRM and VRG, $p < .001$; JTO, $p = .016$; DP-MSRT: RRM and VRG, $p < .001$, JTO, $p = .01$).[3] Comparison of washout-baseline assessment (A_2) with DP-MSRT (BD) showed significant gains in JTO ($p < .001$) and a strong trend for significance in both RRM and VRG ($p = .063$). Intervention with DP-MSRT (BD) was associated with better outcomes than DP-DSLT (BC) (mean increases on the WAB-AQ = 3.2), but differences did not reach statistical significance (Table 3).

Connected speech production

Post-interventions changes in percentage of CIUs relative to baseline (A_1) were variable across patients. Patient RRM improved 14% with DP-DSLT and 70% with DP-MSRT; patient VRG improved 3% with DP-DSLT and 10% with DP-MSRT; and patient JTO decreased 8% with DP-DSLT and improved 13% with DP-MSRT. In patient RRM, who obtained the lower scores in speech production (WAB fluency: 5/10; WAB information content: 7/10) at baseline, remarkable improvements occurred after both interventions, but mostly with DP-MSRT. These improvements were less evident in VRG and JTO who had more fluent and informative verbal productions at baseline (see Tables 1 and 3).

Word and non-word repetition

Baseline scores (A_1) in Word Repetition, Syllable Length from PALPA (test 7) were mildly impaired in two patients (VRG, .88; JTO, .83) and moderately impaired in the other patient (RRM, .71). Word repetition was significantly better than non-word repetition in all three patients at baseline (A_1) (Table 2). As expected, there were no significant changes in single word repetition after both interventions in both patients with mildly impaired performance at baseline (VRG and JTO, $p \geq .25$) most likely due to ceiling effect, whereas a trend for improvement was seen after both interventions in the patient (RRG) with moderately impaired performance (both treatments, $p = .063$). All patients showed moderately impaired ability to repeat items of the Repetition: Non-words PALPA subtest (test 8) at baseline (A_1). Numerically, all patients improved test performance with both interventions. A trend for significant

---

[3] All statistical comparisons were performed using McNemar tests (two-tailed) unless specified.

TABLE 3
Results of language testing at baseline, endpoints and washout

Measure	RRM				VRG				JTO			
	Baseline (Wk 0)	DP/CSLT (Wk 16)	Washout (Wk 20)	DP/MSRT (Wk 28)	Baseline (Wk 0)	DP/CSLT (Wk 16)	Washout (Wk 20)	DP/MSRT (Wk 28)	Baseline (Wk 0)	DP/CSLT (Wk 16)	Washout (Wk 20)	DP/MSRT (Wk 28)
Western aphasia battery (WAB)												
Aphasia quotient (max = 100)[a]	61.6	78.6	77.2	81.6	76	88.4	85	90	79.8	87	76.8	91.1
Picture description												
% Correct information units[b]	13	29	25	83	80	87	77	90	78	70	87	91
Repetition tasks												
Word repetition (n = 24) (PALPA 7)	17	18	17	22	21	23	23	23	20	22	23	23
Non-word repetition (n = 24) (PALPA 8)	8	12	9	12	9	11	8	10	10	14	17	15
Digit production	2	3	3	3	3	3	2	3	3	2	3	3
Word list repetition												
Word pairs												
No delay direct (n = 55)	49	46	46	48	32	52	46	48	30	32	35	38
No delay inverted (n = 55)	45	49	48	48	38	48	45	51	34	38	35	40
Unfilled 5 sec. delay (n = 55)	49	49	48	50	42	50	48	50	25	33	41	43
Triplets (high-frequency) (n = 60)												
Random word combination	0	6	7	12	5	6	6	10	2	4	5	7
Loosely constrained information	2	5	10	12	3	8	8	13	3	7	10	12
Constrained information	5	11	11	17	4	6	10	15	9	15	14	16
Triplets (low-frequency) (n = 60)												
Random word combination	1	8	6	10	0	0	0	9	1	2	4	9
Loosely constrained information	1	8	11	13	0	2	2	10	4	1	5	8
Constrained information	7	8	9	14	1	6	4	10	6	12	6	9
Sentence repetition												
Idiomatic clichés (max = 40)	4	8	6	9	12	15	16	17	17	25	23	24
Novel sentences (max = 40)	11	18	19	23	14	18	15	20	19	27	29	32
Therapy sentences (max 40)	NT	NT	20	39	NT	NT	21	37	NT	NT	22	38
Control sentences (max = 60)	NT	NT	30	44	NT	NT	34	47	NT	NT	35	47

Data from these patients were grouped and treatment effects were analysed using Cohen's d statistic (Cohen, 1988). [a]A₁ (baseline) versus BC (DP-DSLT): Cohen's d = 1.0 and A₂ (washout-baseline) versus BD (DP-MSRT): Cohen's d = 1.2. WAB-AQ: BC (DP-MSLT) versus BD (DP-MSRT), Cohen's d = 1.3. [b]A₁ (baseline) versus BD (DP-MSRT): Cohen's d = 1.14, A₂ (washout-baseline) versus BD (DP-MSRT): Cohen's d = 1.05, BC (DP-CSLT) versus BD (DP-MSRT): Cohen's d = 1.22.
A Cohen's d effect size of .2 to .3 might be a "small" effect, around .5 a "medium" effect and .8 to infinity, a "large" effect (Cohen, 1988).

improvement was only observed in JTO after both interventions ($p = .063$), whereas no changes were found in the remaining two patients.

Digit span

No changes were seen with either therapy in all three patients ($p = .1$) (Table 2).

Word pair repetition

No delay direct. At baseline evaluation, one patient had mildly impaired performance (RRM, .89), whereas the other two patients had moderately impaired performance (VRG, .58; JTO, .54). Patient VRG significantly improved with both DP-DSLT (BC) and DP-MSRT (BD) relative to baseline evaluation (A_1) ($p = .001$), but there were no differences between therapies. His scores in post-washout evaluation (baseline A_2) were significantly better than in baseline evaluation (A_1), and performance after DP-MSRT (BD) were also significantly better than post-washout evaluation (A_2) ($p = .031$). In patient JTO, DP-DSLT (BC) showed a trend for improvement in comparison with baseline (A_1), and a significant improvement with DP-MSRT (BD) was found in comparison with both baseline (A_1) ($p = .008$) and washout-baseline (A_2) evaluations ($p = .031$). No changes were found in patient RRM most likely due to ceiling effect.

No delay inverted. Baseline evaluation revealed that one patient had mildly impaired performance (RRM, .81), whereas the other two patients had moderately impaired performance (VRG, .69; JTO, .61). Patient VRG improved with both DP-DSLT (BC) ($p = .002$) and DP-MSRT (BD) ($p = .001$), but there were no differences between interventions. His scores in washout evaluation (A_2) were significantly better than that in baseline evaluation (A_1) ($p = .016$), and scores after DP-MSRT (BD) were better than those obtained in washout-baseline (A_2) evaluation ($p = .031$). Patient JTO only improved with DP-MSRT (CD) relative to baseline evaluation (A_1) ($p = .008$), and gains with this intervention were significantly better than those obtained with DP-DSLT (BC) ($p = .031$). Scores in this patient also showed a trend for improvement after DP-DSLT (BC) in comparison with baseline evaluation (A_1) ($p = .063$). Patient RRM did not show improvements with either therapy most likely due to ceiling effect.

Unfilled 5-second delay. At baseline evaluation, two patients had mild to moderate impaired performance (RRM, .89; VRG, .76), whereas the other patient had severely impaired performance (JTO, .45). Patient VRG showed significant improvements with both therapies relative to baseline evaluation (A_1), with better scores after DP-MSRT (BD) ($p = .004$) than after DP-DSLT (BC) ($p = .008$). However, there were no differences between these two interventions. In this patient, scores after washout (A_2) were significantly better than those obtained in baseline evaluation (A_1) ($p = .031$). Scores in patient JTO significantly improved with both DP-DSLT (BC) ($p = .008$) and DP-MSRT (BD) ($p = .001$) relative to baseline evaluation (A_1), but gains were significantly better with DP-MSRT (BD) than with DP-DSLT (BC) ($p = .002$). Scores after washout (baseline A_2) were significantly better than those obtained at baseline (A_1) ($p = .001$) and after DP-DSLT (BC) ($p = .008$). No changes were found in patient RRM with either therapy possibly due to ceiling effect.

Word triplet repetition

The number of word triplets repeated accurately by these three patients in each condition is shown in Table 3 and according to serial position in Figure 2. Treatment with DP-DSLT (BC) significantly improved all high-frequency word triplets (Lists 1–3) in comparison with baseline (A_1) in two patients (RRM, $p < .001$; VRG, $p = .008$) but not in the other patient (JTO, $p = .125$). As expected, analyses of all low-frequency word triplets (Lists 4–6) revealed less robust gains than in repetition of high-frequency word strings, but again there were significant improvements with DP-DSLT (BC) relative to baseline (A_1) in two patients (RRM, $p = .031$; VRG, $p = .016$) and no changes in the other patient (JTO, $p = .125$). Comparisons of all high-frequency word triplets (Lists 1–3) between baseline (A_1) and washout (baseline A_2) revealed significantly better performance in post-washout evaluation (A_2) in two patients (RRM, $p < .001$; VRG, $p = .031$). No changes were found in the remaining patient (JTO, $p = .125$). Differences in repetition of all low-frequency word triplets (Lists 4–6) between baseline (A_1) and washout (A_2) revealed significantly better performance in post-washout evaluation (A_2) in one patient (RRM, $p < .001$), a trend for improvement in another (VRG, $p = .063$) and no changes in the remaining patient (JTO, $p = .125$).

After treatment with DP-MSRT (BD) word triplet repetition was significantly better than scores at baseline evaluation (A_1) in all patients in the repetition of both high-frequency strings (Lists 1–3) and low-frequency strings (Lists 4–6) (all patients, $p < .005$). Similar results were found when repetition of high-frequency and low-frequency triplets after treatment with DP-MSRT (BD) was compared with scores

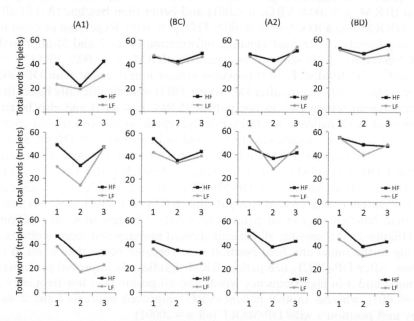

Figure 2. Number of words correctly repeated as function of frequency and serial position in triplets. Graphs depict performance of individual patients (top panel: RRG; medial panel: VRG; and bottom panel: JTO) during repetition of high-frequency (HF) and low-frequency (LF) triplets at baselines (A_1 and A_2) and end points (BC and BD) evaluations. HF triplets included three lists (1, 2 and 3), whereas the remaining three lists (4, 5 and 6) were included in LF triplets. Therefore, the total number of words in each position was 60. See further details in text.

at post-washout testing (A$_2$) in all patients (RRM and VRG, in both measures $p \leq .001$; JTO, in both measures $p = .031$). Importantly, combined intervention with DP-MSRT (BD) significantly improved performance in repetition of high-frequency word triplets in comparison with scores after DP-DSLT (BC) in all patients (both RRM and VRG, $p < .001$; JTO $p = .031$) and in repetition of low-frequency word triplets in two patients (VRG, $p < .001$; JTO $p = .031$). There was a trend for improvement in the remaining patient (RRM, $p = .063$). Finally, results were even more robust when all lists (1–6) were analysed together. Patients' performance with DP-DSLT were significantly better than the ones obtained at baseline (A$_1$) (all patients, $p < .001$) and scores after DP-MSRT were significantly better than those obtained at baseline (A$_1$) and post-washout (A$_2$) testing (all patients in both evaluations, $p < .001$). Scores after DP-MSRT (BD) were better than those obtained with DP-DSLT (BC) (all patients, $p < .001$).

Changes induced by both interventions in the repetition of word triplets were also analysed taking into consideration the semantic relatedness of word strings, so that the following triplets were analysed: random word combination (Lists 1 and 4), loosely constrained information (Lists 2 and 5) and constrained information (Lists 3 and 6). For the sake of simplicity, high-frequency and low-frequency triplets were analysed together. Repetition of word triplets containing random word combination (Lists 1 and 4) improved with DP-DCSL relative to baseline (A$_1$) only in one patient (RRM, $p < .001$). Treatment with DP-MSRT (BD) provided greater improvement than DP-DSLT in two patients (RRM, $p = .008$; VRG, $p < .001$), and a trend for improvement was seen in the remaining patient (JTO, $p = .063$). Scores after DP-MSRT (BD) were significantly better than the ones in washout testing (A$_2$) in two patients (RRM, $p = .004$; VRG, $p < .001$) and better than baseline (A$_1$) in all three patients (RRM and VRG, both $p = .004$; JTO, $p < .008$). Repetition of word triplets containing loosely constrained semantic information (Lists 2 and 5) improved with DP-DCSL relative to baseline in two patients (RRM, $p = .002$; VRG, $p < .016$). Treatment with DP-MSRT (BD) provided greater improvement than DP-DSLT in all patients ($p = .001$). Scores after DP-MSRT (BD) were significantly better than the ones in washout testing (A$_2$) in one patient (VRG, $p < .001$) and also better than baseline (A$_1$) in all patients ($p < .001$). Finally, repetition of word triplets containing constrained semantic information (Lists 3 and 6) improved with DP-DCSL relative to baseline in all patients (RRM and VRG, $p < .016$; JTO, $p < .001$). Treatment with DP-MSRT (BD) provided greater improvement than DP-DSLT two patients (RRM and VRG, $p = .001$). Scores after DP-MSRT (BD) were significantly better than the ones in washout testing (A$_2$) in two patients (RRM and VRG, $p < .001$) and also better than baseline (A$_1$) in all patients ($p < .001$). Changes in serial position were noted (Figure 2). At baseline, all patients showed primacy and recency effects; items occurring in the initial and final position were repeated better than items in medial positions. After DP-DSLT, one patient RRM significantly improved performance in positions 2 and 3 in high-frequency words and all positions in low-frequency words (all, $p < .005$), whereas another patient (VRG) improved positions 1 and 2 with this therapy and position 1 with DP-MSRT (all $p = .0001$).

Clichés and novel sentences

Numerically, all patients showed better baseline performance on repeating novel sentences than clichés although differences did not reach significance. After interventions RRM and VRG did not show improvement in cliché repetition with either intervention, whereas JTO improved his performance in this task with both DP-DSLT (p = .008) and DP-MSRT (p = .016). However, there were no changes when DP-MSRT was compared with washout testing (A_2). As expected, better outcomes were found in repetition of novel sentences in two patients with DP-DSLT compared with baseline (A_1) (RRM, p = .016; JTO, p = .008), and even more robust benefits were found in all three patients when DP-MSRT was compared with baseline (A_1) (RRM and JTO, p <.001; VRG, p = .031). No changes were found, however, when intervention with DP-MSRT was compared with washout testing (A_2).

Therapy and control sentences

Table 3 shows patients' performance on repetition of therapy and control sentences. Scores after DP-MSRT (BD) were significantly better than those obtained at washout (A_2) in all three patients in both therapy sentences (all, p < .005, Fisher Exact Test, two-tailed) and control sentences (all, p <.05, Fisher Exact Test, two-tailed).

DISCUSSION

In this case-series study, we did find that both treatments (DP-DSLT and DP-MSRT) improved repetition of word lists and therapy and control sentences with generalisation of gains to aphasia severity and connected speech during picture description. The combination of DP with MSLT provided better results in connected speech during picture description and word list repetition than DP combined with a less-intensive therapy administered during a longer period (DSLT). Importantly, our patients received the same number of hours (40 hours) of aphasia therapy administered with different timetables (16 weeks of DSLT and 8 weeks of MSRT) and separated between them by a washout period (4 weeks). Furthermore, DSLT trained different language domains (naming, repetition, sentence completion, following commands, spoken object-picture matching and conversations), whereas MSRT trained only a single language domain (sentence repetition). Treatment with DP was safe and well tolerated at usual doses. Only one patient (RRM) developed mild irritability and right leg muscle cramps that not required drug discontinuation. Before advancing further in the discussion, let us examine the theoretical and clinical justification that encouraged us to use MSRT in this case-series study.

DONEPEZIL AND MASSED SENTENCE REPETITION THERAPY

The treatment with MSRT was selected on the basis of previous studies (*see* Introduction) and clinico-anatomical relationships documented in our patients. In the acute stroke period, our three patients had global aphasia secondary to large left perisylvian infarctions. Aphasia severity gradually improved, and when participants were formally evaluated for inclusion in the present trial (mean aphasia duration: 17.3 months), the pattern of language deficits was consistent with the diagnosis of CA (Berthier et al., 2014; Kertesz, 1982; Kohn, 1992). Further baseline cognitive testing of language in these patients revealed impaired/preserved language functions and a pattern of errors (e.g., phonological paraphasias in single word repetition and formal and semantic paraphasias in word list repetition)[4] that placed their syndromes in the *phonological-deep dysphasia* continuum (Jefferies et al., 2007; Martin, 1996; Wilshire & Fisher, 2004). The occurrence of these deficits affecting the storage capacity of phonological and lexical-semantic processes in conjunction with extensive damage involving the left dorsal and ventral auditory streams concurs with the hypothesis suggesting that residual repetition in these disorders reflects partial reliance on right hemisphere activity (Berthier et al., 2012; Demeurisse & Capon, 1991).

Recent studies in Wernicke's aphasics reveal dual acoustic-phonological and semantic breakdowns correlating with left temporo-parietal involvement (Robson, Keidel, Ralph, & Sage, 2012; Robson, Sage, & Lambon Ralph, 2012). Our patients also had lesions involving these posterior cortical sites, yet their baseline performance in certain phonological and lexical-semantic processing tasks ranged from mildly impaired to normal. The mildness of these receptive deficits most likely reflects the consecutive beneficial effect of both spontaneous improvement and aphasia therapy prior to trial inclusion via restitutive integration of non-damaged areas of the left hemisphere, the right hemisphere or both (Fernandez et al., 2004; Harnish et al., 2008; Weiller et al., 1995). Potential candidate regions in the left hemisphere for mediating recovery are the prefrontal-parietal (angular gyrus) cortices (Meltzer, Wagage, Ryder, Solomon, & Braun, 2013; Sharp, Turkheimer, Bose, Scott, & Wise, 2010) and basal ganglia (Harnish et al., 2008). Nevertheless, the role of these areas in recovery cannot be accepted in a straightforward way because patient RRM had partial damage to the prefrontal and angular cortices and all patients had severe damage to areas encompassing the superior longitudinal fasciculus linking these distant cortical sites. The role of left basal ganglia could not be discarded, however, as all patients had only mild involvement of the left putamen and functional neuroimaging in the female CA patient reported by Harnish et al. (2008) with a larger involvement of left basal ganglia, which revealed that she was capable of activating some spared parts of the striatum after massed aphasia therapy. Brain activation after distributed therapy was less noticeable (Harnish et al., 2008). Although functional neuroimaging could not be performed in our patients to examine the spontaneous and treatment-induced compensatory reorganisation of these functions, our findings in anatomical MRI suggest a prominent role of the right hemisphere reorganisation after distributed and massed therapies combined with DP.

We did find that DP-MSRT provided significantly better outcomes than DP-DSLT in most repetition subtests (word pairs, word triplets and novel sentences). Sentences practiced during DP-MSRT also improved, and there was a generalisation of gains to untreated control sentences. We also did find medium to large treatment effects for DP-MSRT in comparison with baselines (A_1, A_2), and DP-CSLT (BC) in aphasia severity (WAB-AQ), and connected speech (%CIUs) with DP-MSRT. Improvement in some of these tasks implies a generalisation of benefits triggered by DP-MSRT, which is in consonance with the results reported in previous intervention studies of CA exclusively treated with repetition training (Kalinyak-Fliszar et al., 2011; Koening-Bruhin & Studer-Eichenberger, 2007; Kohn et al., 1990; Majerus et al., 2005). Nevertheless, findings from the present trial are not fully comparable with previous studies because we augmented the benefits provided by MSRT with a drug. Our findings emphasise the usefulness of implementing neuroscientifically

---

[4] Analysis of errors during word and sentence repetition at baselines (A_1 and A_2) and end points (BC and BD) will be reported elsewhere.

based therapies, like MSRT (and MIT), which are specifically intended to recruit the activity of normal brain structures (right AF) to compensate the function of their homologues in the damaged hemisphere (Schlaug et al., 2009; Zipse et al., 2012).

MECHANISMS UNDERPINNING RECOVERY WITH DONEPEZIL COMBINED WITH MASSED SENTENCE REPETITION THERAPY

Experimental studies in rodents indicate that acetylcholine promotes synaptic transmission, stimulate synaptic plasticity and coordinates the activity of groups of neurons in response to internal and external stimuli eventually enhancing perception, attention, learning and memory processes (Picciotto, Higley, & Mineur, 2012; Sarter et al., 2003, 2005). Cholinergic stimulation in experimental conditions facilitates neuroplasticity, and the resulting changes are more apparent when cholinergic modulation is paired with training (experience-dependent plasticity) (Kleim & Jones, 2008; Sarter et al., 2003, 2005). Human neuroimaging studies of the cholinergic systems substantiate and extend physiological accounts of cholinergic function reported in experimental animal studies (see Bentley, Driver, & Dolan, 2011).

Although we did not perform functional neuroimaging in these three patients, our results invite speculations on the role of DP-MSRT in modulating dysfunctional and underused networks. At baseline, impaired performance on word list and sentence repetition in our patients may be ascribed to synaptic depression in the left lateral cholinergic pathway (insula and fronto-parietal white matter) (Buckingham & Buckingham, 2011; Gotts, Incisa della Rocchetta, & Cipolotti, 2002; Gotts & Plaut, 2004; McNamara & Albert, 2004; Selden, Gitelman, Salamon-Murayama, Parrish, & Mesulam, 1998; Tanaka et al., 2006) with incomplete compensation of deficits by the right perisylvian white matter tracts. We suggest that cholinergic enhancement with DP boosted aphasia therapy effects not only by reverting synaptic depression in dysfunctional areas of the left hemisphere but, more importantly, by recruiting right perisylvian pathways. Recent intervention studies in chronic aphasia demonstrated that benefits in speech production with MIT (Schlaug et al., 2009; Zipse et al., 2012) and in repetition and naming with CIAT (Breier et al., 2011) were associated with functional and structural plasticity of the right AF. We suggest that MSRT (and to a lesser extent DSLT) in combination with DP might also recruit right hemisphere networks. After both treatments, our patients reacquired the ability to repeat with ease previously inaccessible target words in both lists and novel sentences. They also recovered the retention of word order as reflected by significant increment in the number of correct repetition of word triplets and sentences. This may have resulted from reversion of synaptic depression (Gotts & Plaut, 2002) and reduction of spreading activation of competitors (Foster et al., 2012) induced by DP. Also, it is tempting to argue that increased neural efficiency and better task performance promoted by cholinergic stimulation (Ricciardi, Handjaras, Bernardi, Pietrini, & Furey, 2013) were enhanced further with MSRT aimed to strengthen the activity of right hemisphere perisylvian white matter tracts (AF) previously underused in the service of speech repetition. Furthermore, cholinergic enhancement might also have modulated fronto-parietal regions implicated in executive-attentional processes (Demeter & Sarter, 2013) as well as attention and AVSTM through a dynamic interaction between right dorsal and ventral auditory streams (Majerus et al., 2012).

Recovery of production deficits in patients with fluent aphasia generally follows a fixed sequence (e.g., Kertesz, 1984; Kohn, Smith, & Alexander, 1996) evolving from initial production of target-related neologisms, phonological errors and omissions followed by better identifiable phonological and formal errors and eventually progressing to below-average or normal performance. Benefits provided by combined interventions in our three patients were at variance with the usual pattern of recovery from CA described in chronic cases because both interventions circumvented these seemingly obligate steps of recovery. Moreover, we found that DP-MSRT augmented and speeded up recovery in comparison with both DP-DCSLT.

LIMITATIONS

Our intervention trial has the shortcoming of using an open-label, within-subject design implementing two successive treatments. Indeed, one drawback of this design is the increased likelihood of residual beneficial effects of treatment with DP-DSLT on the outcome of DP-MSRT treatment (*carryover* effect) (Grady, Cummings, & Hulley, 2001). Nonetheless, to minimise the impact of the carryover effect on the outcomes of DP-MSRT, we introduced a 4-week washout period between both interventions. Despite the introduction of this non-intervention period, post-washout performance (A_2, week 20) in all patients remained well above the scores obtained at baseline (A_1, week 0). Several hypotheses have been advanced to account for this persistent improvement (Berthier et al., 2003, 2006; Code, Torney, Gildea-Howardine, & Willmes, 2010; FitzGerald et al., 2008; Hughes, Jacobs, & Heilman, 2000), and some of them are related to the use of DP. The first argument maintains that the persistence of gains in cognition after a washout period of 4 weeks may depend on the long plasma half-life of DP (~104 hours) (FitzGerald et al., 2008). Another hypothesis, more compelling than the previous one, suggests that DP promotes brain plasticity in language and short-term memory systems and that these neuroplastic changes persist after DP withdrawal (Berthier et al., 2003, 2006; FitzGerald et al., 2008; Hughes et al., 2000). A complimentary piece of information unrelated to DP treatment refers to the role of delayed beneficial effect of aphasia therapy after its interruption in chronic aphasic patients (Code et al., 2010). It is also worth emphasising in defence of the benefits provided by DP-MSRT that although our patients received the same number of hours of aphasia therapy (40 hours) administered with different timetables, the duration of the drug treatment during DSLT was actually the double (16 weeks) than the one received by patients during MSRT (8 weeks). This suggests that the addition of DP to MSRT increased and speeded up recovery in comparison with DP-DSLT. Finally, our participants' expectation and motivation generated by their participation in a trial with a new pharmacological treatment of aphasia may have played a role in improvement. Even though participants remained motivated throughout the whole trial, in our experience the great expectation for improving depends more on the initial response to pharmacological treatment than the addition of an alternative rehabilitation technique (e.g., MSRT) in the last phase of the trial. Therefore, if our belief is correct, one can expect a greater impact of motivation on outcomes in the initial (DP-DSLT) rather than in final phase (DP-MSRT) of the trial.

REFERENCES

Albert, M. L., Goodglass, H., Helm, N. A., Rubens, A. B., & Alexander, M. P. (1981). Clinical aspects of dysphasia. In G. E. Arnold, F. Winckel, & B. D. Wyke (Eds.), *Disorders of human communication*. New York, NY: Springer-Verlag.

Allen, L., Mehta, S., McClure, J. A., & Teasell, R. (2012). Therapeutic interventions for aphasia initiated more than six months post stroke: A review of the evidence. *Topics in Stroke Rehabilitation, 19*, 523–535.

Arbib, M. A. (2010). Mirror system activity for action and language is embedded in the integration of dorsal and ventral pathways. *Brain and Language, 112*, 12–24.

Ardila, A., & Roselli, M. (1990). Conduction aphasia and verbal apraxia. *Journal of Neurolinguistics, 5*, 1–14.

Asp, A., Cloutier, F., Fay, S., Cook, C., Robertson, M. L., Fisk, J., ... Rockwood, K. (2006). Verbal repetition in patients with Alzheimer's disease who receive donepezil. *International Journal of Geriatric Psychiatry, 21*, 426–431.

Barrett, K. M., Brott, T. G., Brown, Jr., R. D., Carter, R. E., Geske, J. R., Graff-Radford, N. R., . . . Meschia, J. F. Mayo Acute Stroke Trial for Enhancing Recovery (MASTER) Study Group. (2011). Enhancing recovery after acute ischemic stroke with donepezil as an adjuvant therapy to standard medical care: Results of a phase IIA clinical trial. *Journal of Stroke and Cerebrovascular Diseases, 20*, 177–182.

Basso, A. (2003). *Aphasia and its therapy*. New York, NY: Oxford University Press.

Basso, A., Forbes, M., & Boller, F. (2013). Rehabilitation of aphasia. *Handbook of Clinical Neurology, 110*, 325–334.

Basso, A., & Macis, M. (2011). Therapy efficacy in chronic aphasia. *Behavioual Neurology, 24*, 317–325.

Bentley, P., Driver, J., & Dolan, R. J. (2011). Cholinergic modulation of cognition: Insights from human pharmacological functional neuroimaging. *Progress in Neurobiology, 94*, 360–388.

Bernal, B., & Ardila, A. (2009). The role of the arcuate fasciculus in conduction aphasia. *Brain, 132*, 2309–2316.

Berthier, M. L. (2001). Unexpected brain-language relationships in aphasia: Evidence from transcortical sensory aphasia associated with frontal lobe lesions. *Aphasiology, 15*, 99–130.

Berthier, M. L. (2005). Poststroke aphasia: Epidemiology, pathophysiology and treatment. *Drugs and Aging, 22*, 163–182.

Berthier, M. L. (2012). Pharmacological interventions boost language and communication treatment effects in chronic post-stroke aphasia. Presented in the symposium Fortschritte in Neurowissenschaft und Neurorehabilitation der Sprache, 85. Kongress der Deutschen Gesellschaft für Neurologie mit Fortbildungsakademie. Hamburg, Germany, Hauptprogramm, p. 23.

Berthier, M. L., Dávila, G., García-Casares, N., & Moreno-Torres, I. (2014). Post-stroke aphasia. In T. A. Schweizer & R. L. Macdonald (Eds.), *The behavioral consequences of stroke* (pp. 95–117, Chapter 6). New York, NY: Springer Science + Business Media.

Berthier, M. L., Froudist Walsh, S., Dávila, G., Nabrozidis, A., Juárez y Ruiz de Micr, R., Gutiérrez, A., , . . . Garcia-Casares, N. (in press). Dissociated repetition deficits in aphasia can reflect flexible interactions between left dorsal and ventral streams and gender-dimorphic architecture of the right dorsal stream. *Frontiers in Human Neurosciences*.

Berthier, M. L., & Green, C. (2007). Donepezil improves speed and accuracy of information processing in chronic post-stroke aphasia [abstract P01.012]. *Neurology, 68*(Suppl. 1), A10.

Berthier, M. L., Green, C., Higueras, C., Fernández, I., Hinojosa, J., & Martín, M. C. (2006). A randomized, placebo-controlled study of donepezil in poststroke aphasia. *Neurology, 67*, 1687–1689.

Berthier, M. L., Hinojosa, J., Martín, M.del C., & Fernández, I. (2003). Open-label study of donepezil in chronic poststroke aphasia. *Neurology, 60*, 1218–1219.

Berthier, M. L., Lambon Ralph, M. A., Pujol, J., & Green, C. (2012). Arcuate fasciculus variability and repetition: The left sometimes can be right. *Cortex, 48*, 133–143.

Berthier, M. L., & Pulvermüller, F. (2011). Neuroscience insights improve neurorehabilitation of post-stroke aphasia. *Nature Review Neurology, 7*, 86–97.

Berthier, M. L., Pulvermüller, F., Dávila, G., Casares, N. G., & Gutiérrez, A. (2011). Drug therapy of post-stroke aphasia: A review of current evidence. *Neuropsychology Review, 21*, 302–317.

Bhogal, S. K., Teasell, R., & Speechley, M. (2003). Intensity of aphasia therapy, impact on recovery. *Stroke, 34*, 987–993.

Birks, J. (2006). Cholinesterase inhibitors for Alzheimer's disease. *Cochrane Database of Systematic Reviews, 25*(1), CD005593.

Boban, M., Kostovic, I., & Simic, G. (2006). Nucleus subputaminalis: Neglected part of the basal nucleus of Meynert. *Brain, 129*, E42.

Breathnach, C. S. (2011). Jonathan Osborne (1794–1864) and his recognition of conduction aphasia in 1834. *Irish Journal of Medical Sciences, 180*, 23–26.

Breier, J. I., Juranek, J., & Papanicolaou, A. C. (2011). Changes in maps of language function and the integrity of the arcuate fasciculus after therapy for chronic aphasia. *Neurocase, 17*, 506–517.

Buchsbaum, B. R., Baldo, J., Okada, K., Berman, K. F., Dronkers, N., D'Esposito, M., & Hickok, G. (2011). Conduction aphasia, sensory-motor integration, and phonological short-term memory – an aggregate analysis of lesion and fMRI data. *Brain and Language, 119*, 19–28.

Buckingham, H. W., & Buckingham, S. S. (2011). Is recurrent perseveration a product of deafferented functional systems with otherwise normal post-activation decay rates? *Clinical Linguistic and Phonetics, 25*, 1066–1073.

Caplan, D., & Waters, G. (1992). Issues arising regarding the nature and consequences of conduction aphasia. In S. E. Kohn (Ed.), *Conduction aphasia* (pp. 117–149). Hove: Lawrence Erlbaum Associated.

Cappa, S. F., Benke, T., Clarke, S., Rossi, B., Stemmer, B., van Heugten, C. M., . . . European Federation of Neurological Societies. (2005). EFNS guidelines on cognitive rehabilitation: Report of an EFNS task force. *European Journal of Neurology, 12*, 665–680.

Catani, M., Allin, M. P., Husain, M., Pugliese, L., Mesulam, M. M., Murray, R. M., & Jones, D. K. (2007). Symmetries in human brain language pathways correlate with verbal recall. *Proceedings of the National Academy of Sciences USA, 104*, 17163–17168.

Catani, M., Jones, D. K., & Ffytche, D. H. (2005). Perisylvian language networks of the human brain. *Annals of Neurology, 57*, 8–16.

Catani, M., & Mesulam, M. (2008). The arcuate fasciculus and the disconnection theme in language and aphasia: History and current state. *Cortex, 44*, 953–961.

Catani, M., & Thiebaut de Schotten, M. (2012). *Atlas of human brain connections*. New York, NY: Oxford University Press.

Chen, Y., Li, Y. S., Wang, Z. Y., Xu, Q., Shi, G. W., & Lin, Y. (2010). The efficacy of donepezil for post-stroke aphasia: A pilot case control study. *Zhonghua Nei Ke Za Zhi, 49*, 115–118.

Cherney, L. (2012). Aphasia treatment: Intensity, dose parameters, and script training. *International Journal of Speech-Language Pathology, 14*, 424–431.

Cherney, L. R., Erickson, R. K., & Small, S. L. (2010). Epidural cortical stimulation as adjunctive treatment for non-fluent aphasia: Preliminary findings. *Journal of Neurology, Neurosurgery, and Psychiatry, 81*, 1014–1021.

Cherney, L. R., Patterson, J. P., & Raymer, A. M. (2011). Intensity of aphasia therapy: Evidence and efficacy. *Current Neurology and Neuroscience Reports, 11*, 560–569.

Cicerone, K. D., Langenbahn, D. M., Braden, C., Malec, J. F., Kalmar, K., Fraas, M., . . . Ashman, T. (2011). Evidence-based cognitive rehabilitation: Updated review of the literature from 2003 through 2008. *Archives of Physical Medicine and Rehabilitation, 92*, 519–530.

Cloutman, L. L. (2012). Interaction between dorsal and ventral processing streams: Where, when and how? Advance online publication. *Brain and Language*. http://dx.doi.org/10.1016/j.bandl.2012.08.003

Code, C., & Petheram, B. (2011). Delivering for aphasia. *International Journal of Speech and Language Pathology, 13*, 3–10.

Code, C., Torney, A., Gildea-Howardine, E., & Willmes, K. (2010). Outcome of a one month therapy intensive for chronic aphasia: Variable individual responses. *Seminars in Speech and Language, 31*, 21–33.

Cohen, J. (1988). *Statistical power analysis for the behavioural sciences* (2nd ed.). Hillsdale, NJ: Lawrence Erlbaum Associates.

Corballis, M. C. (2010). Mirror neurons and the evolution of language. *Brain and Language, 112*, 25–35.

Cubelli, R., Foresti, A., & Consolini, T. (1988). Reeducation strategies in conduction aphasia. *Journal of Communication Disorders, 21*, 239–249.

Cum, L., & Ellis, A. W. (1999). Why do some aphasics show an advantage on some tests of nonproposi-tional (automatic) speech. *Brain and Language, 70*, 95–118.

De Bleser, R., Cubelli, R., & Luzzatti, C. (1993). Conduction aphasia, misrepresentations, and word representations. *Brain and Language, 45*, 475–494.

Dell, G. S., Martin, N., & Schwartz, M. F. (2007). A case-series test of the interactive two-step model of lexical access: Predicting word repetition from picture naming. *Journal of Memory and Language, 56*, 490–520.

Demeter, E., & Sarter, M. (2013). Leveraging the cortical cholinergic system to enhance attention. *Neuropharmacology, 64*, 294–304.

Demeurisse, G., & Capon, A. (1991). Brain activation during a linguistic task in conduction aphasia. *Cortex, 27,* 285–294.

Dick, A. S., & Tremblay, P. (2012). Beyond the arcuate fasciculus: Consensus and controversy in the connectional anatomy of language. *Brain, 135,* 3529–3550.

Duffau, H., Gatignol, P., Moritz-Gasser, S., & Mandonnet, E. (2009). Is the left uncinate fasciculus essential for language? A cerebral stimulation study. *Journal of Neurology, 256,* 382–389.

Ertelt, D., & Binkofski, F. (2012). Action observation as a tool for neurorehabilitation to moderate motor deficits and aphasia following stroke. *Neural Regeneration Research, 7,* 2063–2074.

Fernandez, B., Cardebat, D., Demonet, J. F., Joseph, P. A., Mazaux, J. M., Barat, M., & Allard, M. (2004). Functional MRI follow-up study of language processes in healthy subjects and during recovery in a case of aphasia. *Stroke, 35,* 2171–2176.

FitzGerald, D. B., Crucian, G. P., Mielke, J. B., Shenal, B. V., Burks, D., Womack, K. B., . . . Heilman, K. M. (2008). Effects of donepezil on verbal memory after semantic processing in healthy older adults. *Cognitive and Behavioral Neurology, 21,* 57–64.

Foster, P. S., Branch, K. K., Witt, J. C., Giovanneti, T., Libon, D., Heilman, K. M., & Drago, V. (2012). Acetylcholinesterase inhibitors reduce spreading activation in dementia. *Neuropsychologia, 50,* 2093–2099.

Francis, D. R., Clark, N., & Humphreys, G. W. (2003). The treatment of an auditory working memory deficit and the implication for sentence comprehension abilities in mild "receptive" aphasia. *Aphasiology, 17,* 723–750.

Fridriksson, J., Hubbard, H. I., Hudspeth, S. G., Holland, A. L., Bonilha, L., Fromm, D., & Rorden, C. (2012). Speech entrainment enables patients with Broca's aphasia to produce fluent speech. *Brain, 135,* 3815–3829.

Friederici, A. D., & Gierhan, S. M. (2013). The language network. *Current Opinion in Neurobiology.* doi: pii:S0959-4388(12)00161-4

Gardner, H. E., Lambon Ralph, M. A., Dodds, N., Jones, T., Ehsan, S., & Jefferies, E. (2012). The differential contributions of pFC and temporo-parietal cortex to multimodal semantic control: Exploring refractory effects in semantic aphasia. *Journal of Cognitive Neuroscience, 24,* 778–793.

Gast, D. L., & Ledford, J. (2009). *Single subject research methodology in behavioral sciences.* Taylor & Francis, e-Library.

Geschwind, N. (1965). Disconnection syndromes in animals and man. *Brain, 88,* 237–294, 585–644.

Geva, S., Correia, M., & Warburton, E. A. (2011). Diffusion tensor imaging in the study of language and aphasia. *Aphasiology, 25,* 543–558.

Gierhan, S. M. (2013). Connections for auditory language in the human brain. *Brain and Language.* doi:pii: S0093-934X(12)00202-7

Gold, B. T., & Kertesz, A. (2001). Phonologically related lexical repetition disorder: A case study. *Brain and Language, 77,* 241–265.

Gotts, S. J., Incisa della Rocchetta, A., & Cipolotti, L. (2002). Mechanisms underlying perseveration in aphasia: Evidence from a single case study. *Neuropsychologia, 40,* 1930–1947.

Gotts, S. J., & Plaut, D. C. (2002). The impact of synaptic depression following brain damage: A connectionist account of "access/refractory" and "degraded-store" semantic impairments. *Cognitive, Affective, & Behavioral Neuroscience, 2,* 187–213.

Gotts, S. J., & Plaut, D. C. (2004). Connectionist approaches to understanding aphasic perseveration. *Seminars in Speech and Language, 25,* 323–334.

Grady, D., Cummings, S. R., & Hulley, S. B. (2001). Designing an experiment: Clinical trials II. In S. B. Huley, S. R. Cummings, W. S. Browner, D. Grady, N. Hearst, & T. B. Newman (Eds.), *Designing clinical research* (pp. 157–174, Chapter 11). Philadelphia, PA: Lippincott Williams & Wilkins.

Gratton, C., Nomura, E. M., Pérez, F., & D'Esposito, M. (2012). Focal brain lesions to critical locations cause widespread disruption of the modular organization of the brain. *Journal of Cognitive Neuroscience, 24,* 1275–1285.

Gvion, A., & Friedmann, N. (2012). Phonological short-term memory in conduction aphasia. *Aphasiology, 26,* 579–614.

Harnish, S. M., Neils-Strunjas, J., Lamy, M., & Eliassen, J. (2008). Use of fMRI in the study of chronic aphasia recovery after therapy: A case study. *Topics in Stroke Rehabilitation, 15*(5), 468–483.

Harvey, D. Y., Wei, T., Ellmore, T. M., Hamilton, C., & Schnur, T. T. (2013). Neuropsychological evidence for the functional role of the uncinate fasciculus in semantic control. *Neuropsychologia, 51,* 789–801.

Hebb, D. O. (1949). *The organization of behavior.* New York, NY: Wiley.

Hickok, G., Houde, J., & Rong, F. (2011). Sensorimotor integration in speech processing: Computational basis and neural organization. *Neuron, 69*, 407–422.

Hickok, G., & Poeppel, D. (2007). The cortical organization of speech processing. *Nature Reviews Neuroscience, 8*, 393–402.

Hong, J. M., Shin, D. H., Lim, T. S., Lee, J. S., & Huh, K. (2012). Galantamine administration in chronic post-stroke aphasia. *Journal of Neurology, Neurosurgery, and Psychiatry, 83*, 675–680.

Hughes, J. D., Jacobs, D. H., & Heilman, K. M. (2000). Neuropharmacology and linguistic neuroplasticity. *Brain and Language, 71*, 96–101.

Husain, M., & Mehta, M. A. (2011). Cognitive enhancement by drugs in health and disease. *Trends in Cognitive Sciences, 15*, 28–36.

Iacoboni, M., Woods, R. P., Brass, M., Bekkering, H., Mazziotta, J. C., & Rizzolatti, G. (1999). Cortical mechanisms of human imitation. *Science, 286*, 2526–2528.

Jefferies, E., Crisp, J., & Lambon Ralph, M. A. (2006). The impact of phonological or semantic impairment on delayed auditory repetition: Evidence from stroke aphasia and semantic dementia. *Aphasiology, 20*, 963–992.

Jefferies, E., Sage, K., & Ralph, M. A. (2007). Do deep dyslexia, dysphasia and dysgraphia share a common phonological impairment? *Neuropsychologia, 45*, 1553–1570.

Junceda, L. (1981). *150 Famosos Dichos del Idioma Castellano*. Madrid: Susaeta Ediciones.

Kalinyak-Fliszar, M., Kohen, F., & Martin, N. (2011). Remediation of language processing in aphasia: Improving activation and maintenance of linguistic representations in (verbal) short-term memory. *Aphasiology, 25*(10), 1095–1131.

Kay, J., Lesser, R., & Coltheart, M. (1992). *Psycholinguistic assessments of language processing in aphasia* (PALPA). Hove: Lawrence Erlbaum Associated.

Kertesz, A. (1982). *The Western aphasia battery*. New York, NY: Grune & Stratton.

Kertesz, A. (1984). Recovery from aphasia. In F. Clifford Rose (Ed.), *Advances in neurology. Volume 42. Progress in aphasiology* (pp. 23–39). New York, NY: Raven Press.

Keysers, C., Kohler, E., Umiltà, M. A., Nanetti, L., Fogassi, L., & Gallese, V. (2003). Audiovisual mirror neurons and action recognition. *Experimental Brain Research, 153*, 628–636.

Kleim, J. A., & Jones, T. A. (2008). Principles of experience-dependent neural plasticity: Implications for rehabilitation after brain damage. *Journal of Speech, Language, and Hearing Research, 51*, S225–S239.

Klein, R. B., & Albert, M. L. (2004). Can drug therapies improve language functions of individuals with aphasia? A review of the evidence. *Seminars in Speech and Language, 25*, 193–204.

Koening-Bruhin, M., & Studer-Eichenberger, F. (2007). Therapy of short-term memory disorders in fluent aphasia: A single case study. *Aphasiology, 21*, 448–458.

Kohler, E., Keysers, C., Umiltà, M. A., Fogassi, L., Gallesse, V., & Rizzolatti, G. (2002). Hearing sounds, understanding actions: Action representation in mirror neurons. *Science, 297*, 846–848.

Kohn, S. E. (1992). *Conduction Aphasia*. Hove: Lawrence Erlbaum Associated.

Kohn, S. E., Smith, K. L., & Alexander, M. P. (1996). Differential recovery from impairment to the phonological lexicon. *Brain and Language, 52*, 129–149.

Kohn, S. E., Smith, K. L., & Arsenault, J. K. (1990). The remediation of conduction aphasia via sentence repetition. *British Journal of Disorders of Communication, 25*, 45–60.

Laska, A. C., Hellblom, A., Murray, V., Kahan, T., & Von Arbin, M. (2001). Aphasia in acute stroke and relation to outcome. *Journal of Internal Medicine, 249*, 413–422.

Lee, J., Fowler, R., Rodney, D., Cherney, L., & Small, S. L. (2010). IMITATE: An intensive computer-based treatment for aphasia based on action observation and imitation. *Aphasiology, 24*, 449–465.

Léger, A., Démonet, J. F., Ruff, S., Aithamon, B., Touyeras, B., Puel, M., . . . Cardebat, D. (2002). Neural substrates of spoken language rehabilitation in an aphasic patient: An fMRI study. *NeuroImage, 17*, 174–183.

López-Barroso, D., Catani, M., Ripollés, P., Dell'acqua, F., Rodríguez-Fornells, A., & de Diego-Balaguer, R. (2013). Word learning is mediated by the left arcuate fasciculus. *Proceedings of the National Academy of Sciences USA, 110*, 13168–13173.

Luria, A., Naydyn, V. L., Tsvetkova, L. S., & Vinarskaya, E. N. (1969). Restoration of higher cortical function following local brain damage. In P. J. Vinken & G. W. Bruyn (Eds.), *Handbook of clinical neurology* (pp. 368–433). Amsterdam: North-Holland.

Majerus, S. (2013). Language repetition and short-term memory: An integrative framework. *Frontiers in Human Neuroscience*. doi:10.3389/fnhum.2013.00357

Majerus, S., Attout, L., D'Argembeau, A., Degueldre, C., Fias, W., Maquet, P., . . . Balteau, E. (2012). Attention supports verbal short-term memory via competition between dorsal and ventral attention networks. *Cerebral Cortex, 22*, 1086–1097.

Majerus, S., van der Kaa, M.-A., Renard, C., Van der Linden, M., & Poncelet, M. (2005). Treating verbal short-term memory deficits by increasing the duration of temporary phonological representations: A case study. *Brain and Language, 95*, 174–175.

Marchina, S., Zhu, L. L., Norton, A., Zipse, L., Wan, C. Y., & Schlaug, G. (2011). Impairment of speech production predicted by lesion load of the left arcuate fasciculus. *Stroke, 42*, 2251–2256.

Martins, I. P., Leal, G., Fonseca, I., Farrajota, L., Aguiar, M., Fonseca, J., . . . Ferro, J. M. (2013). A randomized, rater-blinded, parallel trial of intensive speech therapy in sub-acute post-stroke aphasia: The SP-I-R-IT study. *International Journal of Language and Communication Disorders, 48*, 421–431.

Martin, N. (1996). Models of deep dysphasia. *Neurocase, 2*, 73–80.

Martin, N., & Saffran, E. M. (2002). The relationship of input and output phonological processing: An evaluation of models and evidence to support them. *Aphasiology, 16*, 107–150.

Martin, N., Saffran, E. M., & Dell, G. S. (1994). Recovery in deep dysphasia: Evidence for a relation between auditory-verbal STM capacity and lexical errors in repetition. *Brain and Language, 52*, 83–113.

Martin, N., Saffran, E. M., & Dell, G. S. (1996). Recovery in deep dysphasia: Evidence for a relation between auditory-verbal STM capacity and lexical errors in repetition. *Brain and Language, 52*, 83–113.

McCarthy, R., & Warrington, E. K. (1984). A two-route model of speech production: Evidence from aphasia. *Brain, 107*, 463–485.

McCarthy, R. A., & Warrington, E. K. (1987). The double dissociation of short-term memory for lists and sentences: Evidence from aphasia. *Brain, 110*, 1545–1563.

McNamara, P., & Albert, M. L. (2004). Neuropharmacology of verbal perseveration. *Seminars in Speech and Language, 25*, 309–321.

Meltzer, J. A., Wagage, S., Ryder, J., Solomon, B., & Braun, A. R. (2013). Adaptive significance of right hemisphere activation in aphasic language comprehension. *Neuropsychologia, 51*, 1248–1259

Mesulam, M. M. (2004). The cholinergic innervation of the human cerebral cortex. *Progress in Brain Research, 145*, 67–78.

Mesulam, M. M., Mash, D., Hersh, L., Bothwell, M., & Geula, C. (1992). Cholinergic innervation of the human striatum, globus pallidus, subthalamic nucleus, substantia nigra, and red nucleus. *Journal of Comparative Neurology, 323*, 252–268.

Nadeau, S. E. (2001). Phonology: A review and proposals from a connectionist perspective. *Brain and Language, 79*, 511–579.

Nicholas, L. E., & Brookshire, R. H. (1993). A system for quantifying the informativiness and efficiency of the connected speech of adults with aphasia. *Journal of Speech and Hearing Research, 36*, 338–350.

Nucifora, P. G. P., Verma, R., Melhem, E. R., Gur, R. E., & Gur, R. C. (2005). Leftward asymmetry in relative fiber density of the arcuate fasciculus. *NeuroReport, 16*, 791–794.

Peschke, C., Ziegler, W., Kappes, J., & Baumgaertner, A. (2009). Auditory-motor integration during fast repetition: The neuronal correlates of shadowing. *NeuroImage, 47*, 392–402.

Picciotto, M. R., Higley, M. J., & Mineur, Y. S. (2012). Acetylcholine as a neuromodulator: Cholinergic signalling shapes nervous system function and behaviour. *Neuron, 76*, 116–129.

Pulvermüller, F., & Berthier, M. L. (2008). Aphasia therapy on a neuroscience basis. *Aphasiology, 22*, 563–599.

Pulvermüller, F., Neininger, B., Elbert, T., Mohr, B., Rockstroh, B., Koebbel, P., & Taub, E. (2001). Constraint-induced therapy of chronic aphasia after stroke. *Stroke, 32*, 1621–1626.

Ramanathan, D., Tuszynski, M. H., & Conner, J. M. (2009). The basal forebrain cholinergic system is required specifically for behaviorally mediated cortical map plasticity. *The Journal of Neuroscience, 29*, 5992–6000.

Ricciardi, E., Handjaras, G., Bernardi, G., Pietrini, P., & Furey, M. L. (2013). Cholinergic enhancement reduces functional connectivity and BOLD variability in visual extrastriate cortex during selective attention. *Neuropharmacology, 64*, 305–313.

Rijntjes, M., Weiller, C., Bormann, T., & Musso, M. (2012). The dual loop model: Its relation to language and other modalities. *Frontiers in Evolutionary Neuroscience, 4*, 9. doi:10.3389/fnevo.2012.00009

Robey, R. R. (1998). A meta-analysis of clinical outcomes in the treatment of aphasia. *Journal of Speech, Language, and Hearing Research, 41*, 172–187.

Robson, H., Keidel, J. L., Ralph, M. A., & Sage, K. (2012). Revealing and quantifying the impaired phonological analysis underpinning impaired comprehension in Wernicke's aphasia. *Neuropsychologia, 50*, 276–288.

Robson, H., Sage, K., & Ralph, M. A. (2012). Wernicke's aphasia reflects a combination of acoustic-phonological and semantic control deficits: A case-series comparison of Wernicke's aphasia, semantic dementia and semantic aphasia. *Neuropsychologia, 50*, 266–275.

Rockwood, K., Fay, S., Jarrett, P., & Asp, E. (2007). Effect of galantamine on verbal repetition in AD. A secondary analysis of the VISTA trial. *Neurology, 68*, 1116–1121.

Rorden, C. (2005). MRIcron. Retrieved from http:/www.mccauslandcenter.sc.edu/mricro/mricron

Sage, K., Snell, C., & Lambon Ralph, M. A. (2011). How intensive does anomia therapy for people with aphasia need to be? *Neuropsychological Rehabilitation, 21*, 26–41.

Salis, C. (2012). Short-term memory treatment: Patterns of learning and generalisation to sentence comprehension in a person with aphasia. *Neuropsychological Rehabilitation, 22*, 428–448.

Sarter, M., Bruno, J. P., & Givens, B. (2003). Attentional functions of cortical cholinergic inputs: What does it mean for learning and memory? *Neurobiology of Learning and Memory, 80*, 245–256.

Sarter, M., Hasselmo, M. E., Bruno, J. P., & Givens, B. (2005). Unraveling the attentional functions of cortical cholinergic inputs: Interactions between signal-driven and cognitive modulation of signal detection. *Brain Research Brain Research Reviews, 48*, 98–111.

Saur, D., Kreher, B. W., Schnell, S., Kümmerer, D., Kellmeyer, P., Vry, M. S., . . . Weiller, C. (2008). Ventral and dorsal pathways for language. *Proceeding of the National Academy of Sciences, USA, 105*, 18035–18040.

Schlaug, G., Marchina, S., & Norton, A. (2009). Evidence for plasticity in white-matter tracts of patients with chronic Broca's aphasia undergoing intense intonation-based speech therapy. *Annals of the New York Academy of Sciences, 1169*, 385–394.

Selden, N. R., Gitelman, D. R., Salamon-Murayama, N., Parrish, T. B., & Mesulam, M. M. (1998). Trajectories of cholinergic pathways within the cerebral hemispheres of the human brain. *Brain, 121*, 2249–2257.

Shallice, T., & Warrington, E. K. (1977). Auditory-verbal short-term memory impairment and conduction aphasia. *Brain and Language, 4*, 479–491.

Sharp, D. J., Turkheimer, F. E., Bose, S. K., Scott, S. K., & Wise, R. J. S. (2010). Increased frontoparietal integration after stroke and cognitive recovery. *Annals of Neurology, 68*, 753–756.

Shisler, R. J., Baylis, G. S., & Frank, E. M. (2000). Pharmacological approaches to the treatment and prevention of aphasia. *Aphasiology, 14*, 1163–1186.

Simić, G., Mrzljak, L., Fucić, A., Winblad, B., Lovrić, H., & Kostović, I. (1999). Nucleus subputaminalis (Ayala): The still disregarded magnocellular component of the basal forebrain may be human specific and connected with the cortical speech area. *Neuroscience, 89*, 73–89.

Small, S. L., Buccino, G., & Solodkin, A. (2010). The mirrow neuron system and treatment of stroke. *Developmental Psychobiology, 54*, 293–310.

Small, S. L., & Llano, D. A. (2009). Biological approaches to aphasia treatment. *Current Neurology and Neuroscience Reports, 9*, 443–450.

Song, X., Dornbos, 3rd, D., Lai, Z., Zhang, Y., Li, T., Chen, H., & Yang, Z. (2011). Diffusion tensor imaging and diffusion tensor imaging-fibre tractography depict the mechanisms of Broca-like and Wernicke-like conduction aphasia. *Neurological Research, 33*, 529–535.

Sparks, R., Helm, N., & Albert, M. (1974). Aphasia rehabilitation resulting from melodic intonation therapy. *Cortex, 10*, 303–316.

Stahl, B., Henseler, I., Turner, R., Geyer, S., & Kotz, S. A. (2013). How to engage the right brain hemisphere in aphasics without even singing: Evidence for two paths of speech recovery. *Frontiers in Human Neuroscience, 7*, 35. doi:10.3389/fnhum.2013.00035

Tanaka, Y., Albert, M. L., Fujita, K., Nonaka, C., & Yokoyama, E. (2006). Treating perseverations improves naming in aphasia. *Brain and Language, 99*, 218–219.

Taylor Sarno, M. (1998). Recovery and rehabilitation in aphasia. In M. Taylor Sarno (Ed.), *Acquired aphasia* (pp. 595–619). San Diego, CA: Academic Press.

Ueno, T., Saito, S., Rogers, T. T., & Lambon Ralph, M. A. (2011). Lichtheim 2: Synthesizing aphasia and the neural basis of language in a neurocomputational model of the dual dorsal-ventral language pathways. *Neuron, 72*, 385–396.

Valle, F., & Cuetos, F. (1995). *EPLA: Evaluación del Procesamiento Lingüísticos en la Afasia*. Hove: Lawrence Erlbaum Associates.

Varley, R. (2011). Rethinking aphasia therapy: A neuroscience perspective. *International Journal of Speech-Language Pathology, 13*, 11–20.

Weiller, C., Bormann, T., Saur, D., Musso, M., & Rijntjes, M. (2011). How the ventral pathway got lost: And what its recovery might mean. *Brain and Language, 118*, 29–39.

Weiller, C., Isensee, C., Rijntjes, M., Huber, W., Müller, S., Bier, D., . . . Diener, H. C. (1995). Recovery from Wernicke's aphasia: A positron emission tomographic study. *Annals of Neurology, 37*, 723–732.

Wernicke, C. (1906). Der aphasische Symptomencomplex. In E. von Leyden & F. Klemperer (Eds.), *Die deutsche Klinik am Eingange des 20: Jahrhunderts* (Vol. 6, pp. 487–556)). Berlin: Urban and Schwarzenberg.

Wernicke, C. (1977). *Wernicke's works on aphasia: A sourcebook and review* (pp. 91–145) [Der aphasische Symptomencomplex. Eine psychologische Studie auf anatomischer Basis] (G. H. Eggert, Trans.). New York, NY: Mouton (Original work published 1874).

Whyte, E. M., Lenze, E. J., Butters, M., Skidmore, E., Koenig, K., Dew, M. A., . . . Munin, M. C. (2008). An open-label pilot study of acetylcholinesterase inhibitors to promote functional recovery in elderly cognitively impaired stroke patients. *Cerebrovascular Diseases, 26*, 317–321.

Wilshire, C. E., & Fisher, C. A. (2004). "Phonological" dysphasia: A cross-modal phonological impairment affecting repetition, production, and comprehension. *Cognitive Neuropsychology, 21*, 187–210.

Zipse, L., Norton, A., Marchina, S., & Schlaug, G. (2012). When right is all that is left: Plasticity of right-hemisphere tracts in a young aphasic patient. *Annals of the New York Academy of Sciences, 1252*, 237–245.

Neuroplasticity, neurotransmitters and new directions for treatment of anomia in Alzheimer disease

Adam D. Falchook[1,2], Kenneth M. Heilman[1,2], Glen R. Finney[2], Leslie J. Gonzalez-Rothi[1,2], and Stephen E. Nadeau[1,2]

[1]Malcom Randall Veterans Affairs Medical Center, Gainesville, FL, USA
[2]Department of Neurology and Center for Neuropsychological Studies, University of Florida, Gainesville, FL, USA

Background: Anomia is often one of the earliest signs of Alzheimer disease (AD), and progressive language impairment remains a major source of disability throughout the disease course.
Aims: This article reviews the potential uses of pharmacological adjuvants to augment neuroplasticity during speech and language therapy.
Main Contribution: We begin with a discussion of the nature of anomia in AD from the perspective of classical aphasia models and in terms of a parallel distributed processing model of language. Physiological functions of acetylcholine, norepinephrine and dopamine are reviewed. We consider how pharmacological manipulation of these neurotransmitters in combination with speech and language therapy has the potential to promote maintenance and restoration of the functional connectivity within the lexical, semantic and phonological networks that are the basis of propositional language.
Conclusions: AD is a disease of synaptic loss. People with AD are able to reacquire knowledge, and pharmacological modulation of acetylcholine, norepinephrine and dopamine can influence the maintenance and reformation of neuronal networks.

Partial support for this research is from the Department of Veterans Affairs Office of Research and Development and the State of Florida Department of Elder Affairs. This research was not funded by any other specific grant from any funding agency, commercial organisation or not-for-profit sector. There are no conflicts of interest.

INTRODUCTION

Alzheimer Disease (AD) is characterised by a loss of knowledge and an impaired ability to acquire new knowledge. While prevention of neurodegeneration is central to our search for a cure, for people who suffer from this disease, treatments must also focus on the reacquisition of knowledge that has been considered to be "lost." Recent trials have demonstrated that people with AD are capable of two different types of learning, one based on the re-establishment of connections between substrates for semantics and phonology (Rothi et al., 2009), and the other based on re-establishment of connections in the substrate for semantics (Jelcic et al., 2012). Rothi et al. (2009) also suggested that the concomitant use of donepezil, a centrally acting cholinesterase inhibitor, may have contributed to the capacity for new learning in their participants with AD. Degeneration of neurotransmitter systems, primarily cholinergic neurons (Davies & Maloney, 1976), is central to the pathophysiology of AD. The effects of alterations of neurotransmitter activity must be considered in the context of any strategies to promote re-learning in people with AD. Furthermore, when combined with speech and language therapy, medications that enhance neurotransmitter activity may help maximise the capacity for re-learning in people with AD.

We begin the article with a review of what is known about the nature of anomia in AD. Loss of synaptic connections (the neural instantiation of knowledge) is the essential basis for cognitive impairment in AD (Mazurek & Beal, 1991; Terry et al., 1991). We will first seek to delineate which lost connections are most responsible for anomia. This provides us with a framework to discuss the potential uses of pharmacological adjuvants to leverage neuroplasticity and augment speech and language therapy. We review the neurotransmitter changes in AD, with a focus on acetylcholine, norepinephrine and dopamine and consider how pharmacological modulation of neurotransmitter activity can be used to improve the potential for language rehabilitation.

Geschwind (1967) described differences in pathophysiology between agnosic and aphasic naming errors. Agnosic naming errors result from a disconnection between sensory input and the language network, for example, a disconnection between the visual input from a picture to be named and the language network that mediates production of the name of the picture. Aphasic naming errors result from either a disconnection within the language networks or a degradation of one or more components of these networks. Disorders of these networks may lead to impaired word retrieval and the production of semantically or phonologically related but incorrect names (paraphasic errors), or to complete failure to name (anomia). In some people with AD, naming errors can also be caused by a visual agnosia, most often in the setting of a variant of this disease called posterior cortical atrophy (Benson, Davis, & Snyder, 1988; Levine, Lee, & Fisher, 1993). However, the anomic disorder most often associated with AD is part of a progressive aphasic syndrome.

THE NEUROPSYCHOLOGICAL MECHANISMS OF ANOMIA ASSOCIATED WITH AD

Alois Alzheimer noted that in the course of the disease he first described (1907); there is dissolution of language that begins with anomia and develops into profound impairments of both language comprehension and production of spontaneous speech

(Mathews, Obler, & Albert, 1994). Cummings, Benson, Hill, and Read (1985) studied language in 30 patients with AD and demonstrated that in the earlier stages of the disease, the pattern of language impairment most closely resembled transcortical sensory aphasia, a fluent aphasia with impaired auditory comprehension, anomia and relatively spared ability to repeat. Gorno-Tempini et al. (2008) reported a group of patients with AD who demonstrated language dysfunction characterised by slow speech, word findings pauses, impaired naming and impaired abilities to comprehend and repeat sentences, while the abilities to comprehend and repeat single words were intact or relatively mildly affected. They named this language impairment "progressive logopenic aphasia." Horner, Dawson, Heyman, and Fish (1992) demonstrated that anomic aphasia was the most common taxonomical classification when the Western Aphasia Battery (Kertesz, 1982) was used to assess language in people with AD. This study also demonstrated the limitations of traditional taxonomical aphasia classifications for assessment of language impairment in people with dementia.

Chertkow and Bub (1990) demonstrated that in people with AD, there is a relationship between the loss of ability to name items, loss of ability to identify pictures of named items from among semantically related distracters and loss of ability to answer questions about those items, along with preserved super-ordinate knowledge of those items. Hodges, Patterson, Graham, and Dawson (1996) demonstrated that in patients with minimal, mild and moderate AD, the ability to name pictures significantly correlates with the ability to define the associated names in a way that conveys the "core concept." It was further demonstrated that the features of the definitions that correlated most strongly with the ability to name the associated picture were those aspects of the definition that described physical features of the item. While associative knowledge regarding the items was also lost early in the disease course, this did not correlate with naming ability. Results of this study also demonstrated relative preservation of knowledge of super-ordinate category membership in the mild to moderate stages of AD.

Although the studies discussed above have provided evidence that in AD, anomia is associated with a degradation of semantic knowledge, a loss of semantic knowledge alone may not be sufficient to explain the anomia that develops in the course of AD. Shuren, Geldmacher, and Heilman (1993) reported three patients with AD and sparse spontaneous speech, reduced verbal fluency and an intact ability to name to visual confrontation. Detailed testing of one patient demonstrated that the patient's associative knowledge and semantic knowledge for physical/structural features were both impaired for items that the patient was able to name to visual confrontation. This patient did have an impaired ability to name in response to verbal definition and had impoverished use of content words in spontaneous speech. Thus, preserved semantic knowledge for items may be necessary for use of the items' names in meaningful communication. However, the results of this study suggest a relatively preserved capacity for direct lexical retrieval in response to a visual representation, in the setting of impaired semantic knowledge. Executive functions such as working memory, set shifting, response inhibition and the top–down allocation of attentional resources may also contribute to the lexical retrieval processes necessary to produce a name (Grossman et al., 2004).

Bayles, Tomoeda, Kaszniak, and Trosset (1991) demonstrated that in people with AD, often there was not a consistent pattern of preserved and lost knowledge for individual items when assessed by different semantic tasks and across repeated trials, and performance on semantic knowledge tests varied with task demands. For example, the ability to name a category to which an object belongs was impaired before loss of the ability to name the object, suggesting a basic level effect related to loss of connectivity between the substrates for semantic and phonologic knowledge (e.g., because we use the word "dog" much more often than "mammal," the instantiation of frequency effects in semantic–phonologic connectivity will tend to preserve "dog") (Rogers & McClelland, 2004). The ability to name the object was impaired before loss of the ability to define the object, suggesting loss of connectivity between semantic and phonologic knowledge substrates or loss of connectivity between visual association cortices and the phonological substrate. In the absence of sensory-perceptual agnosia, the loss of ability to define an object suggests loss of semantic knowledge. Thus, these studies imply degradation of connectivity between the semantic and phonologic networks *and* loss of semantic knowledge in AD.

SYNAPTIC DISCONNECTION AND AD

Studies of the language impairments that develop during the course of AD may be most transparently explained by parallel distributed processing (PDP) models of language (Nadeau, 2001). PDP models of language, strongly influenced by the classic Wernicke–Lichtheim diagrams (Heilman, 2006); posit that simultaneous semantic and phonological processing determines word production. This model of parallel semantic and phonological language processing has been supported by results of functional imaging studies in healthy adults (Binder, Medler, Desai, Conant, & Liebenthal, 2005). In people with AD, functional imaging studies have demonstrated alterations in regional brain activation consistent with impairments of both semantic and phonological processing during single word repetition (Peters et al., 2009). These results are consistent with the studies discussed above that demonstrated an impairment of semantic knowledge in AD and the results of a study by Biassou et al. (1995) that demonstrated an impairment of phonological retrieval in AD.

In a PDP model of word production (Nadeau, 2001), the connections between the substrates for semantic and phonological representations provide the basis for naming and constitute the phonological output lexicon (Roth, Nadeau, Hollingsworth, Cimino-Knight, & Heilman, 2006). According to this PDP model, degradation of language ability in AD does not only result from accumulated impairments of distinct systems such as semantics, phonological processing and executive functions. The language dysfunction in AD also reflects, in part, a disconnection between semantic and phonological substrates.

SPEECH AND LANGUAGE THERAPY IN AD

Learning, a form of neuroplasticity, corresponds to changes in connection strengths—synapses in the brain and connection weights in PDP models. The goal of speech and language therapy may be defined as "to maintain and rebuild the connections that comprise the lexicons and semantic knowledge". Chemical neurotransmitters such as acetylcholine, norepinephrine and dopamine have the ability to modify neuronal electrical excitability and to modify the consequences of neuronal depolarisation. In this way, they can influence neuroplasticity, including normal learning. Rothi et al. (2009) and Jelcic et al. (2012) have demonstrated two types of learning that are possible in people with AD.

A recent clinical trial (Rothi et al., 2009) demonstrated the effectiveness of an errorless learning programme (Baddeley & Wilson, 1994; see also Nadeau, Rothi, & Rosenbek, 2008 for a critical review) that trained lexical retrieval without the use of semantic retrieval cues in patients with AD who were being treated with cholinesterase inhibitors. In the first part of each training session, line drawings were presented sequentially and the patient was asked to repeat the names provided by the clinician. During the second part of the training session, the patient was asked to provide the names for the line drawings *only* when the patient felt that she or he knew the correct name. When the patient was not sure of the name for a drawing, the name was provided by the clinician for the patient to repeat. Naming improved in three of the patients, while three patients with more severe dementia did not benefit. The rehabilitation method in this trial facilitated the re-learning of associations between visual and/or semantic representations and the linked phonemic (auditory) and articulomotor representations that together constitute the basis for phonological sequence knowledge and word form. Since all participants in this study received treatment with a cholinesterase inhibitor, the specific effects of this medication on the facilitation of learning could not be directly assessed. However, the study clearly demonstrated that participants with AD were capable of learning and re-establishing the connections between the substrates for visual/semantic and phonological representations.

Jelcic et al. (2012) tested a battery of treatments targeted at improving semantic function in a randomised controlled trial involving 40 participants with very early AD. Half of the participants were assigned to perform tasks that required semantic judgements for words presented in various settings such as lists, sentences and texts. The other half of the participants were assigned to a control treatment that consisted of motor, cognitive and language tasks, but not tasks that explicitly required semantic judgments. Treatment sessions lasting 1 hour were conducted twice weekly for three months. None of the participants received concurrent pharmacotherapy. Participants who received semantic treatment, but not controls, demonstrated improvement on a number of tests that might be expected to benefit from improved semantic function, including the Mini-Mental State Exam (Folstein, Folstein, & McHugh, 1975), tests of naming to confrontation, and both list learning and story recall tests of episodic memory. However, they generally showed little improvement in tests of nonverbal domains. Thus, this study suggests that semantic impairment can be rehabilitated in AD. These two trials provide proof of principle that the major contributors to anomia in AD are susceptible to rehabilitation.

ACETYL CHOLINESTERASE INHIBITORS

Centrally acting cholinesterase inhibitors increase the synaptic levels of acetylcholine, and this is thought to enhance the capacity to learn. Acetylcholine can bind to muscarinic and nicotinic receptors in the brain. When muscarinic receptors bind to acetylcholine, there is activation of GTP-binding proteins and this initiates a cascade of molecular signalling events with diverse outcomes that depend, in part, on the location and subtype of the muscarinic acetylcholine receptor (Levey, 1996). For example, binding of acetylcholine to muscarinic acetylcholine receptors on presynaptic terminals can inhibit the release of excitatory neurotransmitters such as glutamate and aspartate or inhibitory neurotransmitters such as gamma aminobutyric acid (GABA) (Levey, 1996). Activation of presynaptic muscarinic acetylcholine receptors can also lead to feedback inhibition that decreases further release of acetylcholine from the presynaptic terminal (Levey, 1996). Activation of M1 muscarinic receptors expressed at the postsynaptic terminal can increase the neuronal response to N-methyl-D-aspartate, a chemical important for learning and memory (Levey, 1996; Markram & Segal, 1992). Nicotinic acetylcholine receptors include a domain that can bind to acetylcholine or nicotine and a domain that functions as a cation channel that opens in response to binding of acetylcholine or nicotine to the receptor (McKay, Placzek, & Dani, 2007). Activation of nicotinic acetylcholine receptors at the presynaptic terminal can lead to membrane depolarisation, increased levels of intracellular calcium and release of neurotransmitters (McKay, Placzek, & Dani, 2007). Activation of nicotinic acetylcholine receptors at the postsynaptic terminal may increase or decrease the likelihood of achieving long-term potentiation, and this is influenced by the timing relative to stimulation from the presynaptic terminal (Ge & Dani, 2005). Thus, acetylcholine has a central role in processes critical for learning and memory that are mediated by the establishment and maintenance of synaptic connectivity.

Behavioural studies in animal models have demonstrated that acetylcholine plays a critical role in synaptic modification, hence neuroplasticity, including normal learning. Dramatic effects of acetylcholine have been shown on the reorganisation of primary auditory cortex (Kilgard & Merzenich, 1998). Acetylcholine depletion substantially precludes acquisition of a new motor skill (Conner, Culberson, Packowski, Chiba, & Tuszynski, 2003). The central goal of neurorehabilitation is to utilise the brain's capacity for neuroplasticity to facilitate adaptive recovery from neurological disease. Clinical trials in AD have demonstrated a greater benefit from combined treatment with cognitive rehabilitation and a cholinesterase inhibitor, as compared to treatment with a cholinesterase inhibitor alone (Bottino et al., 2005; Chapman, Weiner, Rackley, Hynan, & Zientz, 2004). The study by Rothi et al. (2009) demonstrated that people with AD can rebuild semantic–phonologic connections during an intensive errorless learning rehabilitation programme, and the study by Jelcic et al. (2012) demonstrated that people with AD can rebuild the substrate for semantic knowledge. The animal data, and the results of clinical trials of acetylcholinesterase inhibitors in people with AD, suggest that the capacity of people with AD to learn may be augmented by increasing the levels of acetylcholine in the central nervous system.

Cholinesterase inhibitors were initially proposed as a treatment for AD because of the pathological loss of cholinergic neurons during the course of the disease (Davies & Maloney, 1976). Scopolamine is an anticholinergic medication that has been demonstrated, in healthy adults, to temporarily impair verbal episodic memory, with improvement of this cognitive deficit after administration of a cholinesterase inhibitor (Drachman, 1977). Thus, in addition to the capacity of cholinesterase inhibitors to promote neuroplasticity, it is possible that some of the beneficial effects exerted by this class of medications in people with AD are related to the partial restoration of acetylcholine in the central nervous system. In a 12-week double-blind placebo-controlled study of the centrally acting cholinesterase inhibitor tacrine, patients with mild to moderate AD treated with this medication demonstrated a beneficial effect on naming ability, word finding in spontaneous speech and verbal episodic memory (Farlow et al., 1992). Although tacrine is no longer used clinically because of the concern for hepatic side effects, centrally acting cholinesterase inhibitors (donepezil, galantamine, rivastigmine) are a mainstay in the pharmacological treatment for AD (Cummings, 2004).

In a study by Goldblum et al. (1998), when people with AD were presented with pictures and asked to form semantic associations between the pictures (requiring retrieval of information from semantic memory), subsequent recognition memory for the pictures benefited to a greater extent in those participants with a relatively better ability to correctly perform the semantic association task at the time of memory encoding. This is consistent with the level of processing effect (Craik & Lockhart, 1972), such that recognition of meaning and patterns in a stimulus strengthens the memory trace for that item. FitzGerald et al. (2008) demonstrated that in healthy older adults, donepezil improves immediate and delayed recall for words that are semantically, but not superficially, processed at the time of encoding. The modification of connections within substrates for semantic representations during semantic processing appears to derive significant benefit from the increased levels of acetylcholine associated with administration of cholinesterase inhibitors. Benefit from acetylcholine may be less during superficial processing of the physical features of a stimulus, as this task does not require modification of semantic–semantic connections.

Women and men with AD may respond differently to cholinesterase inhibitors. MacGowan, Wilcock, and Scott (1998) demonstrated that men respond better than women after three months of treatment with the cholinesterase inhibitor tacrine, with response determined by stability or improvement on the Mini-Mental Status Exam (Folstein, Folstein, & McHugh, 1975). This influence of gender on treatment response was not sustained at 12-month follow-up, although of the 68 participants enrolled in the study during the initial three months, only 32 had remained in the study by the time of re-assessment at 12 months. In a double-blind crossover study of 12 people with AD (Davis & Barrett, 2009), men treated with donepezil for two months demonstrated a greater improvement on a test of picture-naming as compared to women treated with this medication for the same duration, with naming re-assessed four months after study initiation.

Anomia rehabilitation programmes often aim to preserve and retrain semantic and semantic–phonological knowledge for target items. Synaptic loss, the impaired ability to form new connections during the course of AD, and the potential benefit associated with the use of a cholinesterase inhibitor should be considered. Future studies are needed to clarify the extent to which semantic and semantic–phonological networks are impaired by cortical degeneration versus cholinergic loss in AD, as the latter may be more amenable to pharmacological intervention. Cholinesterase inhibitors have also been demonstrated to improve naming during recovery from post-stroke aphasia (Berthier et al., 2006; Jacobs et al., 1996; Tanaka, Miyazaki, & Albert, 1997). Although many patients with anomic aphasia have had middle cerebral artery territory infarcts that often do not damage the cholinergic nuclei in the basal forebrain, it is possible that cerebral infarction could de-afferent left fronto-temporo-parietal cortical regions from cholinergic projections.

MEMANTINE

Memantine is thought to act as an N-methyl-D-aspartate (NMDA) receptor antagonist, thereby inhibiting glutamate-mediated excitotoxic death of neurons (Lipton, 2004; Parsons, Stöffler, & Danysz, 2007). There is also evidence that memantine inhibits pathologic phosphorylation of tau (Chohan, Khatoon, Iqbal, & Iqbal, 2006; Li, Sengupta, Haque, Grundke–Iqbal, & Iqbal, 2004). Tau acts to stabilise the polymerised subunits that comprise microtubules, which serve as molecular rails that enable axonal transport. Tau is pathologically hyperphosporylated in AD, making it unavailable to stabilise microtubules and susceptible to polymerisation as neurofibrillary tangles. By inhibiting such hyperphosphorylation, and thereby preserving axonal transport, memantine might help to maintain the integrity of axons and their terminal synapses and perhaps enhance the potential for synaptic modification (learning).

Because NMDA–glutamate ion channel function is essential to normal learning (declarative and procedural), memantine also has the potential to inhibit learning (Dinse, Ragert, Pleger, Schwenkreis, & Tegenthoff, 2003; Schwenkreis, Witscher, Pleger, Malin, & Tegenthoff, 2005). However, in neurological diseases including AD, nonspecific over-activation of NMDA receptors has been proposed to impair learning ability (Parsons, Stöffler, & Danysz, 2007). Memantine blocks excessive NMDA-mediated glutamatergic transmission and this may help restore the normal learning mechanisms (Lipton, 2004). In empirical studies, memantine has been shown to slow the progression of clinical symptoms of AD, either when prescribed as monotherapy (Peskind et al., 2006; Reisberg et al., 2003) or with a cholinesterase inhibitor (Tariot et al., 2004). Furthermore, in a post-hoc analysis of several clinical trials of memantine in people with moderate to severe AD (Ferris et al., 2009), the use of this medication was demonstrated to slow decline on the language component of the Severe Impairment Battery (Panisset, Roudier, Saxton, & Boller, 1994) that was used to assess cognition in these trials. In a trial of treatment of post-stroke aphasia, memantine has been demonstrated to lead to more rapid improvement in language when used as an adjunct to constraint-induced aphasia therapy, with greater responses from the combination of memantine and speech therapy than from either treatment modality alone (Berthier et al., 2009).

CATECHOLAMINES AND AD

Our discussion has focused on the uses of acetylcholinesterase inhibitors and memantine as adjuncts to speech therapy for anomia rehabilitation in people with AD. While cholinesterase inhibitors (donepezil, rivastigmine and galantamine) and the NMDA receptor antagonist memantine are the only medications for treatment of AD approved by the US Food and Drug Administration, there is also evidence for dysfunction of catecholaminergic systems in AD (Cross et al., 1981; Kaddurah–Daouk et al., 2011). Drugs that modulate norepinephrine and dopamine (amphetamines, methylphenidate, levodopa and selective dopamine agonists) are not routinely used for the treatment of AD. However, consideration of the potential roles of these neurotransmitters in language and neuroplasticity can add to our understanding of the nature of language dysfunction in AD and potentially lead to novel therapeutic interventions.

AMPHETAMINES

Dextroamphetamine is a medication that increases the synaptic levels of norepinephrine and dopamine. Studies suggested that administration of dextroamphetamine during rehabilitation therapy hastened recovery and increased the magnitude of recovery from post-stroke hemiplegia (Walker–Batson, Smith, Curtis, Unwin, & Greenlee, 1995) and post-stroke aphasia (Walker-Batson et al., 2001). However, Nadeau and Wu (2006) reviewed the evidence of efficacy of dextroamphetamine as an adjunct to rehabilitation after brain injury and cited a number of methodological problems that afflict essentially all published studies and preclude any firm conclusions about efficacy. Most critically, studies have employed behavioural treatments that had not been proven to be effective in any way, and in the domain of language, have not been shown to generalise to the untrained stimuli probed by outcome measures. If the behavioural treatment does not achieve a reliable neuroplastic effect, there is no effect to be magnified by co-administration of dextroamphetamine. Small language studies are highly susceptible to artefacts of study group heterogeneity. Many studies have had insufficiently long follow-up to determine whether or not there were long-term functional gains associated with use of the medication. Doses of dextroamphetamine that can be used safely in humans are far lower than the doses demonstrated to enhance recovery during the subacute period after a brain injury in animal studies (Feeney, Gonzalez, & Law, 1982).

At doses well tolerated by humans, dextroamphetamine may influence normal learning processes, and there is evidence that this may enhance recovery during the chronic period after a brain injury. Whiting, Chenery, Chalk, and Copland (2007) demonstrated, in a small crossover study of two patients with chronic post-stroke aphasia, that dextroamphetamine, in combination with semantic and phonologic speech therapy, improved naming ability. However, in a placebo-controlled study of four people with chronic nonfluent post-stroke aphasia, Beversdorf et al. (2007) demonstrated that the noradrenergic antagonist propranolol administered at a dose of 40 mg can improve the picture-naming ability. Through its dose-dependent effects on alpha and beta receptors, norepinephrine can amplify or reduce the effects of glutamate on layers II/III and V neurons (sources of intracortical and corticobulbar/corticospinal projections, respectively) (Devilbiss & Waterhouse, 2000). A functional magnetic resonance imaging study has demonstrated that amphetamines lead to increased activation in the primary auditory cortex during a tone-discrimination task and in sensorimotor cortex during a finger-tapping task (Uftring et al., 2001).

Breitenstein et al. (2006a) demonstrated that administration of either amphetamines or levodopa improved the ability of healthy young adults to learn, over 5 days, definitions for 50 pseudowords as trained by association with pictures of real objects. High-impact sprinting has been reported to accelerate acquisition of new verbal information (definitions of pseudowords) and to produce increases in levels of catecholamines and brain-derived neurotrophic factor that correlated with certain measures of learning and retention of the new verbal material (Winter et al., 2007). To the extent permissible with consideration of each patient's comorbidities and physical limitations, the integration of exercise with speech and language rehabilitation programmes may have the potential to enhance neuroplasticity.

To our knowledge, only one study has directly assessed the cognitive effects of dextroamphetamine in people with AD. Lanctôt et al. (2008) demonstrated that people with AD and high levels of apathy did not experience the reward effect from dextroamphetamine that was present in people with AD who had low levels of apathy. This study suggests that frontal–subcortical impairments in some people with AD may influence the response to medications that affect the activity of catecholamines within the central nervous system.

LEVODOPA AND DOPAMINE AGONISTS

Bromocriptine, a dopamine agonist, has been reported to improve language abilities including verbal fluency and lexical retrieval in nonfluent post-stroke aphasia (Albert,

Bachman, Morgan, & Helm-Estabrooks, 1988; Gold, VanDam, & Silliman, 2000; Gupta & Mlcoch, 1992; Raymer et al. 2001; Sabe, Leiguarda, & Starkstein, 1992). However, several clinical trials have not demonstrated benefit from bromocriptine in the treatment of post-stroke aphasia (Gupta, Mlcoch, Scolaro, & Moritz, 1995; Sabe et al., 1995), presenile dementia (Phuapradit, Phillips, Lees, & Stern, 1978), or vascular dementia (Nadeau, Malloy, & Andrew, 1988). These trials that demonstrated no benefit from bromocriptine did not include concurrent speech and language therapy, and it is not known how bromocriptine could augment the response to a structured rehabilitation programme in people with dementia. While Ross and Stewart (1981) demonstrated a beneficial effect of bromocriptine in a patient with akinetic mutism, the different pathophysiology of executive dysfunction in AD may influence the response, or lack of response, to levodopa and dopamine agonists. Akinesia, a lack of spontaneous physical activity, abulia, a lack of spontaneous cognitive activity, and apathy, a lack of emotional investment in physical or cognitive activity, are common features of dementia that can significantly affect quality of life and impair potential for rehabilitation. They are characteristic of frontal–subcortical dysfunction (Heilman, Valenstein, Gonzalez Rothi, & Watson, 2008). The often reduced capacity for self-initiated planning in people with dementia should be taken into account for any rehabilitation programme that involves home practice. Slowed processing speed and impaired set-shifting abilities related to low dopamine levels will affect the optimal rate of presentation of material during rehabilitation sessions.

Sandson and Albert (1987) demonstrated that during naming tests, left hemisphere-damaged stroke patients often respond with the name of a previously named item. They referred to this error type as "recurrent perseveration," and it has been suggested that this may reflect a type of interference by previously retrieved lexical items (McNamara & Albert, 2004). Rothi et al. (2009) noted a reduction in perseverative naming errors during their trial of donepezil combined with errorless learning rehabilitation in AD. Both frontal lobe damage (Luria, 1965) and Parkinson disease (Sandson & Albert, 1987) can impair the ability to inhibit a prepotent motor response. This type of perseveration is known as "stuck in set perseveration." Imamura et al. (1998) demonstrated the potential for bromocriptine to reduce both recurrent perseveration and stuck in set perseveration in a group of patients with vascular or neurodegenerative dementia.

People with AD demonstrate impairments of both semantic activation and attentional processes during semantic priming tasks (Bell, Chenery, & Ingram, 2001). While a semantic concept is often best expressed by a single word, the full comprehension of a semantic concept is often influenced by its diverse associations with other concepts. It is presently unknown how levodopa, dopamine agonists or amphetamines may focus semantic networks in AD and whether or not this would adversely affect neuroplasticity and the ability to rebuild semantic knowledge. Kischka et al. (1996) noted that indirect priming between a prime–target pair such as summer–snow (their example) has been proposed to reflect the spreading of semantic activation from the concepts for summer to winter to snow. In healthy adults, administration of levodopa or pergolide (a D1/D2 dopamine receptor agonist), but not bromocriptine (a selective D2 dopamine receptor agonist), reduces semantic priming between indirectly related entities (Kischka et al., 1996; Roesch-Ely, 2006). These researchers interpreted the observed effects of levodopa and pergolide as "focusing" of semantic networks (Kischka et al., 1996; Roesch-Ely, 2006). Reduction of indirect semantic priming was not demonstrated after administration of the norepinephrine receptor agonist ephedrine (Cios, Miller, Hillier, Tivarus, & Beversdorf, 2009). Administration of levodopa or pergolide may weaken certain diverse connections that contribute to the semantic representation. It is presently not known how focusing of the semantic network may affect lexical retrieval for a concept.

The time required for the spreading of semantic activation has been suggested to explain why indirect priming effects are more prominent at longer stimulus onset asynchronies (the duration between presentation of the prime and the target) (Kischka et al., 1996). However, McKoon and Ratcliff (1992) have provided evidence that priming effects, including "indirect" priming, reflect activation of a direct connection between the prime and the target, although strength of the connection is stronger between words that are more closely related. Bell, Chenery, and Ingram (2001) reviewed evidence that attentional processes, such as the ability to make predictions and to disengage attention from predictions, influence task performance at high but not low stimulus onset asynchronies, and these attentional processes also vary with the relatedness of the prime–target pairs. Thus, dopamine and dopamine agonists that stimulate D1 receptors may focus the activation of semantic networks by reducing the spread of semantic activation from one concept node to the next, by prolonging the time necessary to activate weak semantic connections, and/or by influencing selective attentional processes. A functional imaging study by Copland, McMahon, Silburn, and de Zubicaray (2009) suggested that the effects of levodopa during semantic priming are attributable to a more focused semantic activation of the dominant (most frequently used) meaning of the prime, while semantic representations for less frequently used meanings may be inhibited. Levodopa also appeared to modulate activity in brain regions associated with attentional processes during the task (Copland et al., 2009).

Levodopa is most often used for treatment of Parkinson disease, and Morrison, Borod, Brin, Hälbig, and Olanow (2004) demonstrated that people with moderate to severe Parkinson disease perform better on a confrontation naming test while temporarily "off" medication (levodopa). However, as we have previously discussed, Breitenstein et al. (2006a) demonstrated that administration of either amphetamines or levodopa improved the ability of healthy young adults to learn associations between pseudowords and pictures (semantic concepts). Breitenstein et al. (2006b) also demonstrated that pergolide impaired the ability to form new associations between pseudowords and pictures. Breitenstein et al. (2006b) interpreted these results as attributable to a difference in effect from tonic dopamine receptor stimulation by pergolide and phasic dopamine receptor stimulation by levodopa. Thus, any trial that seeks to use levodopa or a dopamine agonist, with or without concurrent speech therapy, must consider the effects of these medications with regards to executive functions, learning and focusing of semantic network activation. Please also note that the use of pergolide and other ergot dopamine agonists has been significantly limited by the potential for this class of medications to cause valvular heart disease (Schade, Andersohn, Suissa, Haverkamp, & Garbe, 2007; Zanettini et al., 2007).

PRIMUM NON NOCERE

Perhaps of equal or greater importance than the use of pharmacological adjuvants with speech and language rehabilitation is the recognition, and when possible, discontinuation of medications with adverse cognitive side effects in elderly patients with dementia. Many common medications for treatment of allergies, insomnia and urinary incontinence have anticholinergic and antihistaminergic effects that are particularly detrimental to patients with AD (Sunderland et al., 1987). Of the currently available medications for treatment of an overactive bladder (all anticholinergic), darifenacin and trospium appear to have the lowest likelihood of penetrating the blood–brain barrier and there is no evidence of invidious effects of these drugs on cognitive function, most particularly memory (Geller et al., 2012; Kay & Ebinger, 2008; Staskin et al., 2010; Yamada, Kuraoka, Osano, & Ito, 2012). Propranolol, a nonselective beta blocker that crosses the blood–brain barrier, can antagonise some effects of norepinephrine, and while Beversdorf et al. (2007) demonstrated a beneficial effect of propranolol 40 mg on naming in people with chronic nonfluent post-stroke aphaisa, propranolol toxicity has been associated with subacute memory loss (Fisher, 1992). Use of antidopaminergic medications for the treatment of agitation and aggression may potentiate akinesia, abulia and apathy. While antidopaminergic medications should be avoided whenever possible, cholinesterase inhibitors and memantine are potentially effective treatments for the behavioural and psychiatric symptoms associated with AD (Cummings, Schneider, Tariot, Kershaw, & Yuan, 2004; Cummings, Schneider, Tariot, Graham, & Memantine MEM-MD-02 Study Group, 2006), and as such, these medications may also improve the ability to communicate with people with advanced dementia and limited language capacity.

CONCLUSIONS

The challenges inherent in the rehabilitation of language and speech disorders in people with dementia are great, but the demand for effective treatments is far greater. We began with the evidence that AD is a disease of synaptic loss (Mazurek & Beal, 1991; Terry et al., 1991). This is clinically manifest as a loss of connectivity that leads to impairments of semantic knowledge and a degradation of semantic-phonological connections with resultant impairments of speech and language with anomia as an early and prominent feature. Pharmacological modulation of acetylcholine, norepinephrine and dopamine can influence the maintenance and reformation of neuronal networks. The potential of medications that affect these neurotransmitters is likely to be most fully realised when they are administered in combination with speech and language therapies that engage semantic and language networks. Rothi et al. (2009) demonstrated that although lexical-semantic knowledge appears to be lost in people with AD, it can be re-learned. Jelcic et al. (2012) showed that semantic knowledge can be reacquired in people with AD. In the setting of progressive cognitive decline during the course of AD, the capacity to re-learn may be enhanced through pharmacological modulation of neurotransmitters. The use of such pharmacological adjuvants with speech and language therapy will necessarily be a palliative measure to delay progression of disability. Medications that stop the neurodegeneration and synaptic loss will be necessary to achieve a cure. However, unless the disease can be identified and stopped before the onset of cognitive impairment, combined use of speech and language therapy with pharmacological adjuvants that promote neuroplasticity will continue to have considerable potential in the treatment of dementia.

REFERENCES

Albert, M. L., Bachman, D. L., Morgan, A., & Helm-Estabrooks, N. (1988). Pharmacotherapy for aphasia. *Neurology*, *38*, 877–879.

Alzheimer, A. (1907). Über eine eigenartige Erkrankung der Hirnrinde [About a peculiar disease of the cerebral cortex]. *Allgemeine Zeitschrift fur Psychiatrie und Psychisch-Gerichtlich Medizin, 64*, 146–148.

Baddeley, A., & Wilson, B. A. (1994). When implicit learning fails: Amnesia and the problem of error elimination. *Neuropsychologia, 32*, 53–68.

Bayles, K. A., Tomoeda, C. K., Kaszniak, A. W., & Trosset, M. W. (1991). Alzheimer's disease effects on semantic memory: Loss of structure or impaired processing? *Journal of Cognitive Neuroscience, 3*, 166–182.

Bell, E. E., Chenery, H. J., & Ingram, J. C. (2001). Semantic priming in Alzheimer's dementia: Evidence for dissociation of automatic and attentional processes. *Brain and Language, 76*, 130–144.

Benson, D. F., Davis, R. J., & Snyder, B. D. (1988). Posterior cortical atrophy. *Archives of Neurology, 45*, 789–793.

Berthier, M. L., Green, C., Higueras, C., Fernández, I., Hinojosa, J., & Martín, M. C. (2006). A randomized, placebo-controlled study of donepezil in poststroke aphasia. *Neurology, 67*, 1687–1689.

Berthier, M. L., Green, C., Lara, J. P., Higueras, C., Barbancho, M. A., Dávila, G., & Pulvermüller, F. (2009). Memantine and constraint-induced aphasia therapy in chronic poststroke aphasia. *Annals of Neurology, 65*, 577–585.

Beversdorf, D. Q., Sharma, U. K., Phillips, N. N., Notestine, M. A., Slivka, A. P., Friedman, N. M., . . . Hillier, A. (2007). Effect of propranolol on naming in chronic Broca's aphasia with anomia. *Neurocase, 13*, 256–259.

Biassou, N., Grossman, M., Onishi, K., Mickanin, J., Hughes, E., Robinson, K. M., & D'Esposito, M. (1995). Phonologic processing deficits in Alzheimer's disease. *Neurology, 45*, 2165–2169.

Binder, J. R., Medler, D. A., Desai, R., Conant, L. L., & Liebenthal, E. (2005). Some neurophysiological constraints on models of word naming. *Neuroimage, 27*, 677–693.

Bottino, C. M., Carvalho, I. A., Alvarez, A. M., Avila, R., Zukauskas, P. R., Bustamante, S. E., . . . Câmargo, C. H. (2005). Cognitive rehabilitation combined with drug treatment in Alzheimer's disease patients: A pilot study. *Clinical Rehabilitation, 19*, 861–869.

Breitenstein, C., Flöel, A., Korsukewitz, C., Wailke, S., Bushuven, S., & Knecht, S. (2006a). A shift of paradigm: From noradrenergic to dopaminergic modulation of learning? *Journal of the Neurological Sciences, 248*, 42–47.

Breitenstein, C., Korsukewitz, C., Flöel, A., Kretzschmar, T., Diederich, K., & Knecht, S. (2006b). Tonic dopaminergic stimulation impairs associative learning in healthy subjects. *Neuropsychopharmacology, 31*, 2552–2554.

Chapman, S. B., Weiner, M. F., Rackley, A., Hynan, L. S., & Zientz, J. (2004). Effects of cognitive-communication stimulation for Alzheimer's disease patients treated with donepezil. *Journal of Speech Language and Hearing Research: JSLHR, 47*, 1149–1163.

Chertkow, H., & Bub, D. (1990). Semantic memory loss in dementia of Alzheimer's type. What do various measures measure? *Brain, 113*, 397–417.

Chohan, M. O., Khatoon, S., Iqbal, I. G., & Iqbal, K. (2006). Involvement of T2PP2A in the abnormal hyperphorsphorylation of tau and its reversal by memantine. *FEBS Letters, 5680*, 3973–3979.

Cios, J. S., Miller, R. F., Hillier, A., Tivarus, M. E., & Beversdorf, D. Q. (2009). Lack of noradrenergic modulation of indirect semantic priming. *Behavioural Neurology, 21*, 137–143.

Conner, J. M., Culberson, A., Packowski, C., Chiba, A. A., & Tuszynski, M. H. (2003). Lesions of the basal forebrain cholinergic system impair task acquisition and abolish cortical plasticity associated with motor skill learning. *Neuron, 38*, 819–829.

Copland, D. A., McMahon, K. L., Silburn, P. A., & de Zubicaray, G. I. (2009). Dopaminergic neuromodulation of semantic processing: A 4-T FMRI study with levodopa. *Cerebral Cortex, 19*, 2651–2658.

Craik, F. I. M., & Lockhart, R. S. (1972) Levels of processing: A framework for memory research. *Journal of Verbal Learning and Verbal Behavior, 11*, 671–684.

Cross, A. J., Crow, T. J., Perry, E. K., Perry, R. H., Blessed, G., & Tomlinson, B. E. (1981). Reduced dopamine-beta-hydroxylase activity in Alzheimer's disease. *British Medical Journal (Clinical Research Ed), 282*, 93–94.

Cummings, J. L. (2004). Alzheimer's disease. *New England Journal of Medicine, 351*, 56–67.

Cummings, J. L., Benson, F., Hill, M. A., & Read, S. (1985). Aphasia in dementia of the Alzheimer type. *Neurology, 35*, 394–397.

Cummings, J. L., Schneider, L., Tariot, P. N., Kershaw, P. R., & Yuan, W. (2004). Reduction of behavioral disturbances and caregiver distress by galantamine in patients with Alzheimer's disease. *American Journal of Psychiatry, 161*, 532–538.

Cummings, J. L., Schneider, E., Tariot, P. N., Graham, S. M., Memantine MEM-MD-02 Study Group. (2006). Behavioral effects of memantine in Alzheimer disease patients receiving donepezil treatment. *Neurology*, *67*, 57–63.

Davies, P., & Maloney, A. J. (1976). Selective loss of central cholinergic neurons in Alzheimer's disease. *Lancet*, *2*, 1403.

Davis, M. L., & Barrett, A. M. (2009). Selective benefit of donepezil on oral naming in Alzheimer's disease in men compared to women. *CNS Spectrums*, *14*, 175–146.

Devilbiss, D. M., & Waterhouse, B. D. (2000). Norepinephrine exhibits two distinct profiles of action on sensory cortical neuron responses to excitatory synaptic stimuli. *Synapse*, *37*, 273–282.

Dinse, H. R., Ragert, P., Pleger, B., Schwenkreis, P., & Tegenthoff, M. (2003). Pharmacological modulation of perceptual learning and associated cortical reorganization. *Science*, *301*, 91–94.

Drachman, D. A. (1977). Memory and cognitive function in man: Does the cholinergic system have a specific role? *Neurology*, *27*, 783–790.

Farlow, M., Gracon, S. I., Hershey, L. A., Lewis, K. W., Sadowsky, C. H., & Dolan-Ureno, J. (1992). A controlled trial of tacrine in Alzheimer's disease. The Tacrine Study Group. *Journal of the American Medical Association*, *268*, 2523–2529.

Feeney, D. M., Gonzalez, A., & Law, W. A. (1982). Amphetamine, haloperidol, and experience interact to affect rate of recovery after motor cortex injury. *Science*, *217*, 855–857.

Ferris, S., Ihl, R., Robert, P., Winblad, B., Gatz, G., Tennigkeit, F., & Gauthier, S. (2009). Treatment effects of Memantine on language in moderate to severe Alzheimer's disease patients. *Alzheimer's & Dementia, the Journal of the Alzheimer's Association*, *5*, 369–374.

Fisher, C. M. (1992). Amnestic syndrome associated with propranolol toxicity: A case report. *Clinical Neuropharmacology*, *15*, 397 403.

FitzGerald, D. B., Crucian, G. P., Mielke, J. B., Shenal, B. V., Burks, D., Womack, K. B., . . . Heilman, K. M. (2008). Effects of donepezil on verbal memory after semantic processing in healthy older adults. *Cognitive and Behavioral Neurology*, *21*, 57–64.

Folstein, M. F., Folstein, S. E., & McHugh, P. R. (1975). "Mini-mental state". A practical method for grading the cognitive state of patients for the clinician. *Journal of Psychiatric Research*, *12*, 189–198.

Ge, S., & Dani, J. A. (2005). Nicotinic acetylcholine receptors at glutamate synapses facilitate long-term depression or potentiation. *Journal of Neuroscience*, *25*, 6084–6091.

Geller, E. J., Crane, A. K., Wells, E. C., Robinson, B. L., Jannelli, M. L., Khandelwal, C. M., . . . Busby-Whitehead, J. (2012). Effect of anticholinergic use for the treatment of overactive bladder on cognitive function in postmenopausal women. *Clinical Drug Investigations*, *32*, 697–705.

Geschwind, N. (1967). The varieties of naming errors. *Cortex*, *3*, 97–112.

Gold, M., VanDam, D., & Silliman, E. R. (2000). An open-label trial of bromocriptine in nonfluent aphasia: A qualitative analysis of word storage and retrieval. *Brain and Language*, *74*, 141–156.

Goldblum, M. C., Gomez, C. M., Dalla Barba, G., Boller, F., Deweer, B., Hahn, V., & Dubois, B. (1998). The influence of semantic and perceptual encoding on recognition memory in Alzheimer's disease. *Neuropsychologia*, *36*, 717–729.

Gorno-Tempini, M. L., Brambati, S. M., Ginex, V., Ogar, J., Dronkers, N. F., Marcone, A., . . . Miller, B. L. (2008). The logopenic/phonological variant of primary progressive aphasia. *Neurology*, *71*, 1227–1234.

Grossman, M., McMillan, C., Moore, P., Ding, L., Glosser, G., Work, M., & Gee, J. (2004). What's in a name: Voxel-based morphometric analyses of MRI and naming difficulty in Alzheimer's disease, frontotemporal dementia and corticobasal degeneration. *Brain*, *127*, 628–649.

Gupta, S. R., & Mlcoch, A. G. (1992). Bromocriptine treatment of nonfluent aphasia. *Archives of Physical Medicine and Rehabilitation*, *73*, 373–376.

Gupta, S. R., Mlcoch, A. G., Scolaro, C., & Moritz, T. (1995). Bromocriptine treatment of nonfluent aphasia. *Neurology*, *45*, 2170–2173.

Heilman, K. M. (2006). Aphasia and the diagram makers revisited: An update of information processing models. *Journal of Clinical Neurology*, *2*, 149–162.

Heilman, K. M., Valenstein, E., Gonzalez Rothi, L. J., & Watson, R. T. (2008). Upper limb action-intentional and cognitive-apraxic motor disorders. In W. G. Bradley, R. B. Daroff, G. M. Fenichel, & J. Jankovic (Eds.), *Neurology in Clinical Practice*. (5th ed., pp. 2320–2325). Philadelphia, PA: Butterworth Heinemann Elsevier.

Hodges, J. R., Patterson, K., Graham, N., & Dawson, K. (1996). Naming and knowing in dementia of Alzheimer's type. *Brain and Language*, *54*, 302–325.

Horner, J., Dawson, D. V., Heyman, A., Fish, A. M. (1992). The usefulness of the Western Aphasia Battery for differential diagnosis of Alzheimer dementia and focal stroke syndromes: Preliminary evidence. *Brain and Language*, *42*, 77–88.

Imamura, T., Takanashi, M., Hattori, N., Fujimori, M., Yamashita, H., Ishii, K., & Yamadori, A. (1998). Bromocriptine treatment for perseveration in demented patients. *Alzheimer Disease and Associated Disorders*, *12*, 109–113.

Jacobs, D., Shuren, J., Gold, M., Adair, J. C., Bowers, D., Williamson, D. G., & Heilman, K. M. (1996). Physostigmine pharmacotherapy for anomia. *Neurocase*, *2*, 83–91.

Jelcic, N., Cagnin, A., Menghello, F., Turolla, A., Ermani, M., & Dam, M. (2012). Effects of lexical-semantic treatment on memory in early Alsheimer disease: An observer-blinded randomized controlled trial. *Neurorehabilitation and Neural Repair*, *26*, 949–956.

Kaddurah-Daouk, R., Rozen, S., Matson, W., Han, X., Hulette, C. M., Burke, J. R., . . . Welsh-Bohmer, K. A. (2011). Metabolomic changes in autopsy-confirmed Alzheimer's disease. *Alzheimers Dementia*, *7*, 309–317.

Kay, G. G., & Ebinger, U. (2008). Preserving cognitive function for patients with overactive bladder: Evidence for a differential effect with darifenacin. *International Journal of Clinical Practice*, *62*, 1792–1900.

Kertesz, A. (1982). *Western Aphasia Battery*. New York, NY: Grune & Stratton.

Kilgard, M. P., Merzenich, & M. M. (1998). Cortical map reorganization enabled by nucleus basalis activity. *Science*, *279*, 1714–1718.

Kischka, U., Kammer, T., Maier, S., Weisbrod, M., Thimm, M., & Spitzer, M. (1996). Dopaminergic modulation of semantic network activation. *Neuropsychologia*, *34*, 1107–1113.

Lanctôt, K. L., Herrmann, N., Black, S. E., Ryan, M., Rothenburg, L. S., Liu, B. A., & Busto, U. E. (2008). Apathy associated with Alzheimer disease: Use of dextroamphetamine challenge. *American Journal of Geriatric Psychiatry*, *16*, 551–557.

Levey, A. I. (1996). Muscarinic acetylcholine receptor expression in memory circuits: Implications for treatment of Alzheimer disease. *Proceedings of the National Academy of Science USA*, *93*, 13541–13546.

Levine, D. N., Lee, J. M., & Fisher, C. M. (1993). The visual variant of Alzheimer's disease: a clinicopathologic case study. *Neurology*, *43*, 305–313.

Li, L., Sengupta, A., Haque, N., Grundke-Iqbal, I., & Iqbal, K. (2004). Memantine inhibits and reverses the Alzheimer type abnormal hyperphosphorylation of tau and associated neurodegeneration. *FEBS Letters*, *566*, 261–269.

Lipton, S. A. (2004). Paradigm shift in NMDA receptor antagonist drug development: Molecular mechanism of uncompetitive inhibition by memantine in the treatment of Alzheimer's disease and other neurologic disorders. *Journal of Alzheimer's Disease: JAD*, *6*, S61–S74.

Luria, A. R. (1965). Two kinds of motor perseveration in massive injury of the frontal lobes. *Brain*, *88*, 1–10.

MacGowan, S. H., Wilcock, G. K., & Scott, M. (1998). Effect of gender and apolipoprotein E genotype on response to anticholinesterase therapy in Alzheimer's disease. *International Journal of Geriatric Psychiatry*, *13*, 625–630.

Markram, H., & Segal, M. (1992). The inositol 1,4,5-trisphosphate pathway mediates cholinergic potentiation of rat hippocampal neuronal responses to NMDA. *Journal of Physiology*, *447*, 513–533.

Mathews, P. J., Obler, L. K., & Albert, M. L. (1994). Wernicke and Alzheimer on the language disturbances of dementia and aphasia. *Brain and Language*, *46*, 439–462.

Mazurek, M. F., & Beal, M. F. (1991). Cholecystokinin and somatostatin in Alzheimer's disease postmortem cerebral cortex. *Neurology*, *41*, 716–719.

McKay, B. E., Placzek, A. N., & Dani, J. A. (2007). Regulation of synaptic transmission and plasticity by neuronal nicotinic acetylcholine receptors. *Biochemical Pharmacology*, *74*, 1120–1133.

McNamara, P., & Albert, M. L. (2004). Neuropharmacology of verbal perseveration. *Semininars in Speech and Language*, *25*, 309–321.

McKoon, G., & Ratcliff, R. (1992). Spreading activation versus compound cue accounts of priming: Mediated priming revisited. *Journal of Experimental Psychology: Learning, Memory, and Cognition*, *18*, 1155–1172.

Morrison, C. E., Borod, J. C., Brin, M. F., Hälbig, T. D., & Olanow, C. W. (2004). Effects of levodopa on cognitive functioning in moderate-to-severe Parkinson's disease (MSPD). *Journal of Neural Transmission*, *111*, 1333–1341.

Nadeau, S. E. (2001). Phonology: A review and proposals from a connectionist perspective. *Brain and Language*, *79*, 511–579.

Nadeau, S. E., Malloy, P. F., & Andrew, M. E. (1988). A crossover trial of bromocriptine in the treatment of vascular dementia. *Annals of Neurology*, *24*, 270–272.

Nadeau, S. E., Rothi, L. J. G., & Rosenbek, J. C. (2008). Language rehabilitation from a neural perspective. In: R. Chapey (Ed.), *Language Intervention Strategies in Aphasia and Related Neurogenic Communication Disorders* (5th ed., pp. 689–734). Philadelphia, PA: Lippincot Williams & Wilkins.

Nadeau, S. E., & Wu, S. S. (2006). CIMT as a behavioral engine in research on physiological adjuvants to neurorehabilitation: The challenge of merging animal and human research. *NeuroRehabilitation, 21*, 107–130.

Panisset, M., Roudier, M., Saxton, J., & Boller, F. (1994). Severe impairment battery: A neuropsychological test for severely demented patients. *Archives of Neurology, 51*, 41–45.

Parsons, C. G., Stöffler, A., & Danysz, W. (2007). Memantine: A NMDA receptor antagonist that improves memory by restoration of homeostasis in the glutamatergic system—too little activation is bad, too much is even worse. *Neuropharmacology, 53*, 699–723.

Peskind, E. R., Potkin, S. G., Pomara, N., Ott, B. R., Graham, S. M., Olin, J. T., & McDonald, S. (2006). Memantine treatment in mild to moderate Alzheimer disease: A 24-week randomized, controlled trial. *American Journal of Geriatric Psychiatry, 14*, 704–715.

Peters, F., Majerus, S., Collette, F., Degueldre, C., Del Fiore, G., Laureys, S., . . . Salmon, E. (2009). Neural substrates of phonological and lexicosemantic representations in Alzheimer's disease. *Human Brain Mapping, 30*, 185–199.

Phuapradit, P., Phillips, M., Lees, A. J., & Stern, G. M. (1978). Bromocriptine in presenile dementia. *British Medical Journal, 1*, 1052–1053.

Raymer, A. M., Bandy, D., Adair, J. C., Schwartz, R. L., Williamson, D. J., Gonzalez Rothi, L. J., & Heilman, K. M. (2001). Effects of bromocriptine in a patient with crossed nonfluent aphasia: A case report. *Archives of Physical Medicine and Rehabilitation, 82*, 139–144.

Reisberg, B., Doody, R., Stöffler, A., Schmitt, F., Ferris, S., Möbius, H. J. (2003). Memantine in moderate-to-severe Alzheimer's disease. Memantine Study Group. *New England Journal of Medicine, 348*, 1333–1341.

Roesch-Ely, D., Weiland, S., Scheffel, H., Schwaninger, M., Hundemer, H. P., Kolter, T., & Weisbrod, M. (2006). Dopaminergic modulation of semantic priming in healthy volunteers. *Biological Psychiatry, 60*, 604–611.

Rogers, T. T., & McClelland, J. L. (2004). *Semantic cognition. parallel distributed processing approach.* Cambridge, MA: MIT Press.

Ross, E. D., & Stewart, R. M. (1981). Akinetic mutism from hypothalamic damage: successful treatment with dopamine agonists. *Neurology, 31*, 1435–1439.

Roth, H. L., Nadeau, S. E., Hollingsworth, A. L., Marie Cimino-Knight, A., & Heilman, K. M. (2006). Naming concepts: Evidence of two routes. *Neurocase, 12*, 61–70.

Rothi, L. J., Fuller, R., Leon, S. A., Kendall, D., Moore, A., Wu, S. S., . . . Nadeau, S. E. (2009). Errorless practice as a possible adjuvant to donepezil in Alzheimer's disease. *Journal of the International Neuropsychological Society, 15*, 311–322.

Sabe, L., Leiguarda, R., & Starkstein, S. E. (1992). An open-label trial of bromocriptine in nonfluent aphasia. *Neurology, 42*, 1637–1638.

Sabe, L., Salvarezza, F., García Cuerva, A., Leiguarda, R., & Starkstein, S. (1995). A randomized, double-blind, placebo-controlled study of bromocriptine in nonfluent aphasia. *Neurology, 45*, 2272–2274.

Sandson, J., & Albert, M. L. (1987). Perseveration in behavioral neurology. *Neurology, 37*, 1736–1741.

Schade, R., Andersohn, F., Suissa, S., Haverkamp, W., & Garbe, E. (2007). Dopamine agonists and the risk of cardiac-valve regurgitation. *New England Journal of Medicine, 356*, 29–38.

Schwenkreis, P., Witscher, K., Pleger, B., Malin, J. P., & Tegenthoff, M. (2005). The NMDA antagonist memantine affects training induced motor cortex plasticity—a study using transcranial magnetic stimulation. *BMC Neuroscience, 6*, 35.

Shuren, J., Geldmacher, D., & Heilman, K. M. (1993). Nonoptic aphasia: Aphasia with preserved confrontation naming in Alzheimer's disease. *Neurology, 43*, 1900–1907.

Staskin, D., Kay, G., Tannenbaum, C., Goldman, H. B., Bhashi, K., Ling, J., & Oefelein, M. G. (2010). Trospium chloride has no effect on memory testing and is assay undetectable in the central nervous system of older patients with overactive bladder. *International Journal of Clinical Practice, 64*, 1294–1230.

Sunderland, T., Tariot, P. N., Cohen, R. M., Weingartner, H., Mueller III, E. A., & Murphy, D. L. (1987). Anticholinergic sensitivity in patients with dementia of the Alzheimer type and age-matched controls. A dose-response study. *Archives of General Psychiatry, 44*, 418–426.

Tanaka, Y., Miyazaki, M., & Albert, M. L. (1997). Effects of increased cholinergic activity on naming in aphasia. *Lancet, 350*, 116–117.

Tariot, P. N., Farlow, M. R., Grossberg, G. T., Graham, S. M., McDonald, S., Gergel, I., Memantine Study Group. (2004). Memantine treatment in patients with moderate to severe Alzheimer disease already receiving donepezil: A randomized controlled trial. *Journal of the American Medical Association, 291,* 317–324.

Terry, R. D., Masliah, E., Salmon, D. P., Butters, N., DeTeresa, R., Hill, R., . . . Katzman, R. (1991). Physical basis of cognitive alterations in Alzheimer's disease: Synapse loss is the major correlate of cognitive impairment. *Annals of Neurology, 30,* 572–580.

Uftring, S. J., Wachtel, S. R., Chu, D., McCandless, C., Levin, D. N., & de Wit, H. (2001). An fMRI study of the effect of amphetamine on brain activity. *Neuropsychopharmacology, 25,* 925–935.

Walker-Batson, D., Curtis, S., Natarajan, R., Ford, J., Dronkers, N., Salmeron, E., . . . Unwin, D. H. (2001). A double-blind, placebo-controlled study of the use of amphetamine in the treatment of aphasia. *Stroke, 32,* 2093–2098.

Walker-Batson, D., Smith, P., Curtis, S., Unwin, H., & Greenlee, R. (1995). Amphetamine paired with physical therapy accelerates motor recovery after stroke. Further evidence. *Stroke, 26,* 2254–2259.

Whiting, E., Chenery, H. J., Chalk, J., & Copland, D. A. (2007). Dexamphetamine boosts naming treatment effects in chronic aphasia. *Journal of the International Neuropsychological Society, 13,* 972–979.

Winter, B., Breitenstein, C., Mooren, F. C., Voelker, K., Fobker, M., Lechtermann, A., . . . Knecht, S. (2007). High impact running improves learning. *Neurobiolgy of Learning and Memory, 87,* 597–609.

Yamada, S., Kuraoka, S., Osano, A., & Ito, Y. (2012). Characterizationn of bladder selectivity of antimuscarinic agents on the basis of *in vivo* drug-receptor binding. *International Neurourology, 16,* 107–115.

Zanettini, R., Antonini, A., Gatto, G., Gentile, R., Tesei, S., & Pezzoli, G. (2007). Valvular heart disease and the use of dopamine agonists for Parkinson's disease. *New England Journal of Medicine, 356,* 39–46.

Effects of memantine treatment on language abilities and functional communication: A review of data

Michael Tocco[1], Kathryn Bayles[2], Oscar L. Lopez[3],
Robert K. Hofbauer[1], Vojislav Pejović[4], Michael L. Miller[4],
and Judith Saxton[3]

[1]Forest Research Institute, Harborside Financial Center, Jersey City, NJ, USA
[2]Department of Communication Sciences and Disorders, University of Central Arkansas, Conway, AR, USA
[3]Department of Neurology, University of Pittsburgh, Pittsburgh, PA, USA
[4]Prescott Medical Communications Group, Chicago, IL, USA

Background: Impairment in language abilities occurs in a number of neurological conditions, including Alzheimer's disease (AD) and other dementias, primary progressive aphasia, multiple sclerosis and stroke. Currently, no pharmacotherapy is approved for aphasia of any aetiology. Memantine, an antagonist of *N*-methyl-D-aspartate glutamate receptors that is approved for the treatment of moderate-to-severe AD, has shown promising results on several measures of language and communication in clinical trials.
Aims: This review summarises the knowledge gathered from prospective studies and *post hoc* analyses involving patients with AD and other neurological conditions in whom the effects of memantine treatment on language or communication have been examined.
Main Contribution: PubMed searches yielded a total of four prospective studies and three *post hoc* analyses that assessed the effects of memantine on language and communication in AD (one additional *post hoc* analysis was published as a conference proceeding

The authors wish to thank Torrey Volkman, Rebecca Myers, Mark Domke and Bill Sterling of Prescott Medical Communications Group, Chicago, IL for assistance with literature searches, checking of outlines and drafts for accuracy and consistency and creation of figures.

This study was sponsored by Forest Research Institute (FRI), a subsidiary of Forest Laboratories, Inc., the US marketer of memantine. Dr Saxton has received consulting fees from FRI for assistance in developing study MEM-MD-71, cited in this review. In addition, Dr Saxton received support from FRI for travel to meetings, and payments from H Lundbeck A/S (an international marketer of memantine) for lectures at company-sponsored symposia. Finally, Dr Saxton receives royalties from sales of the Severe Impairment Battery (SIB), a psychiatric assessment scale discussed in this review. Dr Bayles receives royalties from the sale of the Functional Linguistic Communication Inventory (FLCI), a communication test discussed in this review. Dr Lopez has served as a consultant for Lundbeck, Eli Lilly, Baxter and Merz Pharma, an international marketer of memantine. Drs Hofbauer and Tocco are employees of FRI and Drs Miller and Pejović are employees of Prescott Medical Communications Group, a paid consultant and medical communications contractor of FRI.

only), together with seven prospective studies in other conditions (Parkinson's disease, frontotemporal lobe degeneration, chronic post-stroke aphasia, primary progressive aphasia, multiple sclerosis, risk of dementia). Available data suggest that memantine provides modest language and communication benefits in patients with moderate-to-severe AD; potential benefits in Parkinson's disease and post-stroke aphasia were also observed. *Conclusions*: Memantine may provide clinical benefits in language and communication in AD and other neurological conditions. Since communication problems create a significant burden for patients and their caregivers, larger prospective trials, conducted to provide more precise estimates of benefits in that domain, are merited.

Impairment in language abilities occurs in a number of neurological conditions, including Alzheimer's disease (AD) (Ahmed, de Jager, Haigh, & Garrard, 2012) and other dementias (Reilly, Rodriguez, Lamy, & Neils-Strunjas, 2010; Zec et al., 1999), primary progressive aphasia (Gorno-Tempini et al., 2011; Mesulam, 2003), multiple sclerosis (Ghezzi, Goretti, Portaccio, Roscio, & Amato, 2010) and stroke (Saur & Hartwigsen, 2012). Currently, the treatment of aphasia, regardless of its aetiology, is primarily focused on intensive language-action therapy, such as constraint-induced aphasia therapy (Berthier, 2005; Pulvermüller & Berthier, 2008). Although no pharmacotherapy is currently approved for aphasia, trials involving drugs that target dopaminergic (bromocriptine), cholinergic (donepezil, bifemelane), GABAergic (piracetam, zolpidem) or dopaminergic-serotonergic-catecholaminergic pathways (dexanfetamine, moclobemide) have been conducted with mixed results (Berthier, 2005; Portugal Mda, Marinho, & Laks, 2011; Pulvermüller & Berthier, 2008). Currently, it is not clear whether a single drug can provide benefits for language impairment across multiple aetiologies.

Communication impairment has been studied extensively in patients with AD, and there is some evidence for the improvement of communication-related symptoms with pharmacotherapy (see below). Difficulties with language appear early in AD and increase with disease progression (Verma & Howard, 2012); deficits in spontaneous word finding, confrontation naming and verbal fluency (Bayles, Tomoeda, Cruz, & Mahendra, 2000; Forstl & Kurz, 1999; Honig & Mayeux, 2001) are commonly observed, as well as impairment in functional communication (Fromm & Holland, 1989). Language-related symptoms in patients with AD are frequently associated with increased caregiver stress and burden (Ripich, 1994).

Memantine, a drug approved for the treatment of moderate-to-severe AD (2007; McShane, Areosa Sastre, & Minakaran, 2006), is an uncompetitive, voltage dependent NMDA receptor antagonist with fast on/off binding kinetics that blocks pathological, tonic glutamate influx without interfering with normal, activity-generated glutamatergic signalling (Parsons, Danysz, & Quack, 1999; Parsons, Stoffler, & Danysz, 2007). Because of these properties, memantine has the potential to interrupt glutamate-mediated neurotoxic cascades that have been proposed to underlie a wide variety of neuropathological conditions. NMDA receptors have also been implicated in processes such as the lateralisation of language (Ocklenburg et al., 2011) and the development of autism spectrum disorders (Chez et al., 2007; Choudhury, Lahiri, & Rajamma, 2012), so it is conceivable that glutamatergic pathways may also influence receptive or expressive language, and that memantine could play an as yet undetermined role in the alleviation of language impairment. Memantine has also been shown to bind nicotinic acetylcholine receptors and serotonin receptors, albeit with a lower affinity (Parsons et al., 2007), and to affect other neuronal processes such as tau phosphorylation (Francis, 2009), although it is not clear what role, if any, these effects may have on language. Preclinical studies have also demonstrated an efficacy for memantine in models of depression and anxiety, either of which may also affect speech production, although clinical studies investigating these indications have produced conflicting results (Parsons et al., 1999; Sani et al., 2012).

Post hoc analyses of clinical trial data from patients with AD (Emre, Mecocci, & Stender, 2008; Ferris et al., 2009b; Mecocci, Bladstrom, & Stender, 2009; Pomara, Ott, Peskind, & Resnick, 2007; Schmitt, van Dyck, Wichems, & Olin, 2006; Tocco & Graham, 2010), as well as anecdotal clinical reports, have suggested that memantine treatment may be associated with improvements in language and communication abilities. These observations led investigators to prospectively examine the effect of memantine on communication in patients with moderate-to-severe AD (Grossberg et al., 2013; Saxton et al., 2012; Schulz et al., 2011), Parkinson's disease dementia (Litvinenko, Odinak, Mogil'naya, & Perstnev, 2010), post-stroke aphasia (Berthier et al., 2009) and other conditions.

This review summarises the knowledge gathered from prospective studies and *post hoc* analyses involving patients with AD and other neurological conditions in whom the effects of memantine treatment on language or communication have been examined. It should be noted that most of the studies were either small prospective trials or *post hoc* analyses of larger trials, some of which have only been published in the form of abstracts at scientific meetings, and several of the outcome measures were exploratory or not validated specifically in patients with language impairment. Therefore, this review was designed to provide a broad overview of the available literature, rather than a full systematic analysis.

METHODS

Data collection

The PubMed database was searched on 20 December 2012, for relevant records using a search criterion of "memantine AND (language OR communication OR aphasia)", which yielded 61 titles. Nine of those 61 titles were considered relevant, i.e., constituted reports on memantine trials or *post hoc* analyses in AD and other conditions that examined language-related items. Additional studies were identified by examining lists of "related publications" generated by PubMed in response to the search strategy and by examining references cited in the selected publications. We focused on trials that assessed language production, as opposed to those that assessed mental faculties involved in language processing (e.g., verbal learning and memory). Finally, authors included their own previous reports if deemed relevant by author consensus, including conference proceedings that have not yet been published as peer-reviewed manuscripts. All authors reviewed the initial PubMed search results and agreed on the final list of publications and reports.

RESULTS

Alzheimer's disease

The largest studies evaluating the effects of memantine on communication have been performed in patients with moderate-to-severe AD (defined as having a score of <20 on the Mini-Mental State Examination [MMSE; Folstein, Folstein, &

McHugh, 1975]). Several randomised, double-blind, placebo-controlled trials in this patient population have included measures that can be used to assess language and functional communication, either directly and prospectively, or indirectly using *post hoc* analyses (see Table 1). All of the *post hoc* analyses reported here used data pooled from two or more of the randomised trials shown in Table 1, although the specific populations that were combined and the assessment tools that were applied depended upon the year that the analyses were performed, the availability of study data and the group that performed each analysis.

Communication parameters examined in post hoc analyses of randomised clinical trials. Several *post hoc* analyses investigating the effects of memantine on language and communication have used data pooled from four large 6-month, randomised, double-blind, placebo-controlled trials (Grossberg et al., 2013; Reisberg et al., 2003; Tariot et al., 2004; van Dyck, Tariot, Meyers, & Resnick, 2007). All four trials (see Table 1) were conducted in patients with moderate-to-severe AD, who had baseline MMSE scores <15. In one pooled analysis of these trials, language items from the *Severe Impairment Battery* (SIB) (Panisset, Roudier, Saxton, & Boller, 1994; Schmitt et al., 1997), were combined in a face-valid manner to create three language subscales (see Figure 1): **Naming** (15 items; 28 points), **Reading/Writing** (4 items; 8 points) and **Comprehension/Repetition/Discourse** (4 items; 8 points) (Tocco & Graham, 2010).

After 6 months of treatment, memantine-treated patients showed significantly less decline than placebo-treated patients on all three subscales (see Figure 2) (Tocco & Graham, 2010).

In a separate *post hoc* analysis, Mecocci et al. (2009) pooled data from all participants from three randomised trials of memantine in moderate-to-severe AD (MMSE <15) (Reisberg et al., 2003; Tariot et al., 2004; van Dyck et al., 2007), and patients with moderate AD (MMSE 10–19) from three randomised trials in mild-to-moderate AD (Bakchine & Loft, 2008; Peskind et al., 2006; Porsteinsson, Grossberg, Mintzer, & Olin, 2008). In this analysis, the language domain from the SIB (moderate-to-severe AD trials) and language items from the *Alzheimer's Disease Assessment Scale—cognitive subscale* (ADAS–cog; mild-to-moderate AD trials) (Rosen, Mohs, & Davis, 1984) were analysed separately. After 6 months, memantine-treated patients with moderate-to-severe AD demonstrated significantly less decline than placebo-treated patients on the SIB language domain (highlighted items from Figure 1 plus item 6; 46 points total), with significant benefits observed as early as Week 4 (observed cases [OC] analysis, $p < .05$) (Mecocci et al., 2009). In the less severely affected patients from the mild-to-moderate AD trials, significant benefits for memantine compared with placebo were also observed after 24 weeks on the ADAS–cog language items of commands (OC; $p < .001$) and comprehension ($p < .05$), but not on items of language, object naming, word recall, word finding or word recognition (Mecocci et al., 2009). This suggests that the benefits of memantine may be greater in patients with more advanced disease.

A similar analysis (Emre et al., 2008), which included the same subset of patients as the study by Mecocci et al. (2009), combined the ADAS–cog and SIB items into clusters representing language, memory and praxis. The language cluster contained the ADAS–cog items of object naming, commands, language, comprehension and word finding (25 points), as well as SIB language items (46 points). After 24 weeks, a significantly higher percentage of memantine-treated than placebo-treated patients demonstrated an improvement on the language cluster, and a significantly lower

TABLE 1

Memantine phase III/IV trials in AD

Condition	Study	Trial design, duration, size	Treatment	Language-related efficacy parameters[a]	Significance at endpoint: MEM vs. PBO[b]
Trials used in post hoc analyses of language and communication					
Moderate to Severe AD (MMSE: 3–14)	MRZ-9001-9605 (Reisberg et al., 2003) NCT not available	RDBPC 28 weeks $N = 252$ PBO: 126 MEM: 126	10 mg BID MEM PBO	SIB (s)	SIB: $p < .001$
Moderate to Severe AD (MMSE: 5–14)	MEM-MD-01 (van Dyck et al., 2007) NCT not available	RDBPC 24 weeks $N = 350$ PBO: 172 MEM: 178	10 mg BID MEM PBO	ADCS–ADL$_{19}$ (p) SIB (p) BGP (s)	ADCS–ADL$_{19}$: $p = .28$ SIB: $p = .616$ BGP: $p = .197$
Moderate to Severe AD (MMSE: 5–14)	MEM-MD-02 (Tariot et al., 2004) NCT not available	RDBPC 24 weeks $N = 403$ PBO/DON: 201 MEM/DON: 202	10 mg BID MEM PBO	ADCS–ADL$_{19}$ (p) SIB (p) BGP (s)	ADCS–ADL$_{19}$: $p = .03$ SIB: $p < .001$ BGP: $p = .001$
Moderate to Severe AD (MMSE: 5–14)	IE-2101 (Kitamura et al., 2011) NCT not available	RDBPC 24 weeks $N = 315$ PBO: 108 MEM 10 mg: 107 MEM 20 mg: 100	10 mg QD 20 mg QD MEM PBO	ADCS–ADL-J (p) SIB-J (p)	ADCS–ADL-J: $p = .838$[c] SIB-J: $p = .005$[c]
Mild to Moderate AD (MMSE: 10–22)	MEM-MD-10 (Peskind et al., 2006) NCT not available	RDBPC 24 weeks $N = 403$ PBO: 202 MEM: 201	10 mg BID MEM PBO	ADAS–cog (p) ADCS–ADL$_{23}$ (s)	ADAS–cog: $p = .003$; ADCS–ADL$_{23}$: $p = .89$

(Continued)

TABLE 1
(Continued)

Condition	Study	Trial design, duration, size	Treatment	Language-related efficacy parameters[a]	Significance at endpoint: MEM vs. PBO[b]
Mild to Moderate AD (MMSE: 10–22)	MEM-MD-12 (Þorsteinsson et al., 2008) NCT not available	RDBPC 24 weeks $N = 433$ PBO: 216 MEM: 217	20 mg QD MEM PBO	ADAS–cog (p) ADCS–ADL$_{23}$ (s)	ADAS–cog: $p = .184$ ADCS–ADL$_{23}$: $p = .816$
Mild to Moderate AD (MMSE: 11–23)	99679 (Bakchine & Loft, 2008) NCT not available	RDBPC 24 weeks $N = 470$ PBO: 152 MEM: 318	10 mg BID MEM PBO	ADAS–cog (p) ADCS–ADL$_{23}$ (s)	ADAS–cog: $p = .156$ ADCS–ADL$_{23}$: $p = .912$
Trials in which language and communication were studied prospectively					
Mild to Moderate AD (MMSE: 15–23)	MEM-MD-15 (Weiner et al., 2011) NCT00334906	Exploratory, single-arm, delayed start, OL 48 weeks (Weeks 1–24, ChEI-only; Weeks 25–48, MEM-ChEI) $N = 47$	10 mg BID MEM	BNT	BNT: $p = .038$
Moderate AD (MMSE: 10–19)	MEM-MD-71 (Saxton et al., 2012) NCT00469456	RDBPC 12 weeks $N = 265$ PBO: 129 MEM: 136	10 mg BID MEM PBO	FLCI (p) ASHA FACS (s) OPT (o)	FLCI: $p = .070$ ASHA FACS: $p = .022$ OPT: $p = .189$
Moderate to Severe AD (MMSE: 3–14)	MEM-MD-50 (Grossberg et al., 2013) NCT00322153	RDBPC 24 weeks $N = 677$ PBO/ChEI: 335 MEM/ChEI: 342	28 mg QD MEM (extended release) PBO	SIB (p) VFT (o)	SIB: $p = .001$ VFT: $p = .004$

(*Continued*)

TABLE 1
(Continued)

Condition	Study	Trial design, duration, size	Treatment	Language-related efficacy parameters[a]	Significance at endpoint: MEM vs. PBO[b]
Moderate to Severe AD (MMSE: <20)	MRZ 90001-0608/1 (Schulz et al., 2011) NCT0624026	OL 16 weeks $N = 97$	20 mg QD MEM	FLCI (s) ADCS–ADL$_{19}$ (s) VFT (s)	CERAD–NP: $p < .0001$[d] FLCI: $p < .0001$[d] ADCS–ADL$_{19}$: $p = .4459$[d] VFT: $p = .0036$[d]

The studies listed in this table are clinical trials that either were prospectively designed to investigate the effects of memantine on measures of language and communication, or that utilised primary (p), secondary (s), or other (o) outcomes with communication-related components that were later analysed. p-Values indicate the significance of the original trial outcomes.

AD = Alzheimer's disease; ADAS–cog = Alzheimer's Disease Assessment Scale—cognitive subscale; ADCS–ADL$_{19}$ = the 19-item Alzheimer's Disease Cooperative Study-Activities of Daily Living scale; ADCS–ADL$_{23}$ = the 23-item Alzheimer's Disease Cooperative Study–Activities of Daily Living scale; ADCS–ADL-J = the Alzheimer's Disease Cooperative Study–Activities of Daily Living Inventory Japanese version; ASHA FACS = the combined Social Communication and Communication of Basic Needs subscales of the American Speech-Language-Hearing Association Functional Assessment of Communication Skills for Adults scale; BGP = the Behavioural Rating Scale for Geriatric Patients; BID = twice-daily dosing; BNT = Boston Naming Test; CERAD–NP = Consortium to Establish a Registry for Alzheimer's Disease–Neuropsychological Battery; ChEI = cholinesterase inhibitor; DON = donepezil; FLCI = the Functional Linguistic Communication Inventory; MEM = memantine; NCT = National Clinical Trial registration number; OL = open label; OPT = Oral Production Task; PBO = placebo; QD = once-daily dosing; RDBPC = randomised, double-blind, placebo-controlled; SIB = Severe Impairment Battery; SIB-J = Severe Impairment Battery-Japanese version; VFT = Verbal Fluency Test.

[a] Measures of global condition were not included because they are not specifically language-related; however, the contribution of communication to a patient's global condition may be notable.

[b] Data shown are LOCF, except where primary publications reported only OC data.

[c] Comparison was between PBO and 20 mg MEM.

[d] Change from baseline at endpoint.

Item		Points			Item		Points		
1a	Shake hands	2	1	0	20	Confrontation naming-spoon	2	1	0
1b	Follow directions	2	1	0	21	Using spoon-photo	2	1	0
1c	Sit here	2	1	0	22	Object naming-spoon	2	1	0
2	Examiner's name	2	1	0	23	Using object-spoon	2	1	0
3	Patient's name	2	1	0	24	Forced choice naming-spoon		1	0
4a	Write name	2	1	0	25	Object immediate	2	1	0
4b	Copy name	2	1	0	26	Color naming-blue	2	1	0
5	Month	2	1	0	27	Color matching	2	1	0
6	Months of year	2	1	0	28	Colored block	2	1	0
7	City	2	1	0	29	Color discrimination	2	1	0
8a	Responsive naming-cup	2	1	0	30a	Color naming-red	2	1	0
8b	Responsive naming-spoon	2	1	0	30b	Color naming-green	2	1	0
9a	Reading comprehension	2	1	0	30c	Shape identification-square	2	1	0
9b	Verbal comprehension	2	1	0	31	Shape matching	2	1	0
9c	Reading	2	1	0	32	Shape-remembers square	2	1	0
10	Sentence	2	1	0	33	Shape discrimination	2	1	0
11a	Saying 'People spend money'	2	1	0	34a	Shape identification-circle	2	1	0
11b	Saying 'Baby'	2	1	0	34b	Shape identification-triangle	2	1	0
12	Digit span	2	1	0	35a	Drawing-circle	2	1	0
13	Fluency	2	1	0	35b	Drawing-square	2	1	0
14	Examiner's name-delayed	2	1	0	36	Auditory span	2	1	0
15	Confrontation naming-cup	2	1	0	37	Visual span	2	1	0
16	Using cup-photo	2	1	0	38	Object delayed (cup/spoon)	2	1	0
17	Object naming-cup	2	1	0	39	Orienting to name	2	1	0
18	Using object-cup	2	1	0	40	Free discourse	2	1	0
19	Forced choice naming-cup		1	0					

Naming subscale items
Reading/Writing subscale items
Comprehension/Repetition/Discourse subscale items

Figure 1. Severe Impairment Battery language items and subscales (Panisset et al., 1994; Schmitt et al., 1997, 2006; Tocco et al., 2008).

percentage of memantine-treated patients worsened on the measure, using both OC and a last observation carried forward (LOCF) approach for imputation of missing data (see Figure 3) (Emre et al., 2008).

A separate group performed a similar analysis (Ferris et al., 2009a), in which they created a new scale (*SIB-L*) based on 21 language-related SIB items that were selected through a principal components factor analysis. In a sample of 801 patients with MMSE scores <15, pooled from the three aforementioned trials of memantine in moderate-to-severe AD (Reisberg et al., 2003; Tariot et al., 2004; van Dyck et al., 2007) and a Japanese trial (Kitamura, Honma, Nakamura, & Yoshimura, 2011), memantine-treated patients performed significantly better on the SIB-L than placebo-treated patients after 6 months ($p = .0182$) (Ferris et al., 2009b). In addition, in the subset of patients with marked language impairment at baseline (SIB-L score, ≤20), significantly more memantine-treated patients than placebo-treated patients experienced a clinically relevant improvement (defined as a score increase greater than 3.7 points) after 6 months (25.4% vs. 10.8%; $p = .041$), and significantly fewer

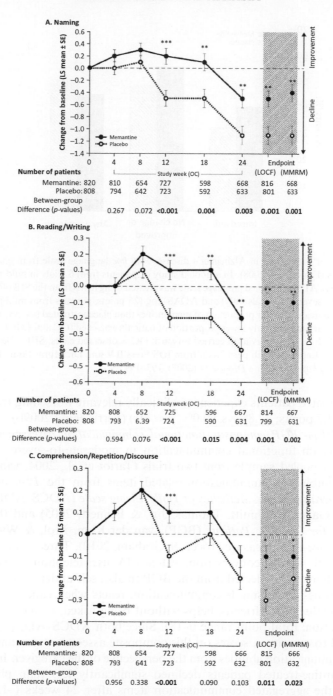

Figure 2. Effects of memantine in Alzheimer's disease: Severe Impairment Battery language subscales (Tocco & Graham, 2010). Patients with AD who were treated with memantine for 24 weeks demonstrated significantly less decline than placebo-treated patients on Severe Impairment Battery subscales that evaluate Naming (15 items; 28 points), Reading/Writing (4 items; 8 points) and Comprehension/Repetition/Discourse (4 items; 8 points). ADAS–cog = Alzheimer's Disease Assessment Scale—cognitive subscale; LOCF = last observation carried forward; LS = least squares; MMRM = mixed-effects model with repeated measures; OC = observed cases; SE = standard error. *$p < .05$; **$p < .01$; ***$p < .001$; bold p-values indicate those attaining statistical significance.

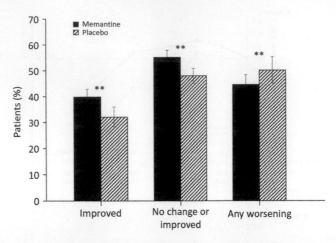

Figure 3. Effects of memantine in Alzheimer's disease: *Post hoc* language scale from combined SIB and ADAS–cog items (Emre et al., 2008). In a pooled study of patients from 6 trials in mild-to-moderate and moderate-to-severe AD, a combined language scale was created using items from the SIB (46 points, patients from moderate-to-severe AD trials only) and ADAS–cog (25 points, patients from mild-to-moderate AD trials only). A significantly higher proportion of memantine- than placebo-treated patients improved on this language scale, while a significantly lower proportion of patients worsened (OC and LOCF analyses; LOCF shown here). LOCF = last observation carried forward; OC = observed cases; SIB = Severe Impairment Battery. **$p < .01$. Reprinted with permission from IOS Press B.V. and Dr. Murat Emre. Figure originally published in *Journal of Alzheimer's Disease 14* (2008), 193–199.

memantine-treated patients experienced clinically relevant worsening (score decrease greater than 3.7 points; 32.8% vs. 60.0%, $p = .01$) (Ferris et al., 2009b).

ADCS-ADL₁₉- BGP composite functional communication assessment. The effect of memantine on functional communication in moderate-to-severe AD was also examined in a pooled sample from two trials (Tariot et al., 2004; van Dyck et al., 2007), by combining communication-related items from the *19-item Alzheimer's Disease Cooperative Study–Activities of Daily Living scale* (ADCS–ADL$_{19}$) (Galasko et al., 1997; Galasko, Schmitt, Thomas, Jin, & Bennett, 2005) and the *Behavioral Rating Scale for Geriatric Patients* (BGP) (van der Kam, Mol, & Wimmers, 1971) into a single face-valid measure (Tocco & Graham, 2010). Three items were selected from the ADCS–ADL$_{19}$ (conversation, watches TV, uses telephone; total point range 0–12) and 9 items were selected from the BGP (makes self understood, knows family and friend names, understands communication, reacts when called by name, keeps occupied, socialises with friends, helps without being asked, cooperative and enters into conversation; total point range 0–18). Since both ADCS–ADL$_{19}$ and BGP are administered to caregivers, scores on this composite assessment presumably reflect a patient's communication abilities from the perspective of the caregiver. In this analysis (OC), memantine-treated patients declined significantly less than placebo-treated patients on the aggregated communication items after 24 weeks (-1.2 ± 0.21 vs. -0.3 ± 0.20, $p = .004$, respectively; LS mean difference $\pm$ standard error), suggesting that caregivers can also detect memantine-related advantages in communication (Tocco & Graham, 2010).

Communication parameters examined prospectively. In part due to the promising results from the post hoc analyses discussed above, several memantine trials in AD were prospectively designed to include measures of language and communication as

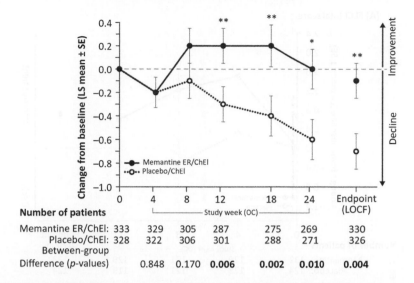

Figure 4. The effect of extended-release memantine on verbal fluency in patients with moderate-to-severe Alzheimer's disease (Grossberg et al., 2013). Treatment with extended-release memantine provided significant benefits on verbal fluency in patients with moderate-to-severe AD who were already taking a ChEI. The verbal fluency score is the number of items from a category (animals) that the patient can name in 1 minute. ChEI = cholinesterase inhibitor; LOCF = last observation carried forward; LS = least squares; OC = observed cases; SE = standard error. *$p < .05$; **$p < .01$; bold p-values indicate those attaining statistical significance. © Reprinted with kind permission from Springer Science+Business Media B.V. Figure originally published in *CNS Drugs* (2013), 27(6), 469–478 by Grossberg et. al.

efficacy parameters (Grossberg et al., 2013; Saxton et al., 2012; Schulz et al., 2011; Weiner et al., 2011), including two trials that were designed for the specific purpose of assessing the effects of memantine on language and communication (Saxton et al., 2012; Schulz et al., 2011) (see Table 1).

In a trial of extended-release memantine in patients with moderate-to-severe AD receiving stable acetylcholinesterase inhibitor therapy (Grossberg et al., 2013), memantine treatment was associated with significantly less decline in semantic verbal fluency (animal naming) compared with placebo treatment, as assessed using the *Verbal Fluency Test* of semantic memory (Isaacs & Kennie, 1973; Morris et al., 1989) at Weeks 12, 18 and 24 (see Figure 4) (Grossberg et al., 2013).

One prospective, randomised, double-blind, placebo-controlled trial was designed to investigate the effects of memantine on functional communication in patients with moderate AD (MMSE: 10–19) (Saxton et al., 2012). In this trial, functional communication was assessed by means of the *Functional Linguistic Communication Inventory* (FLCI; primary efficacy parameter; total score of 87 points) (Bayles & Tomoeda, 1994) and the combined subscales of Social Communication and Communication of Basic Needs from the *American Speech-Language-Hearing Association Functional Assessment of Communication Skills for Adults* (ASHA-FACS; secondary parameter; total score of 196 points) (Frattali, Thompson, Holland, Wohl, & Ferketic, 1995). Compared with the placebo group, patients who received memantine showed significant improvement on the FLCI (see Figure 5A) at Week 4 (LOCF and OC, $p = .028$) and Week 8 (LOCF, $p = .015$; OC, $p = .023$) and a numerical (non-significant) improvement at study endpoint (Week 12; LOCF, $p = .070$; OC, $p = .184$); a mixed-effects model with repeated measures (MMRM) analysis of

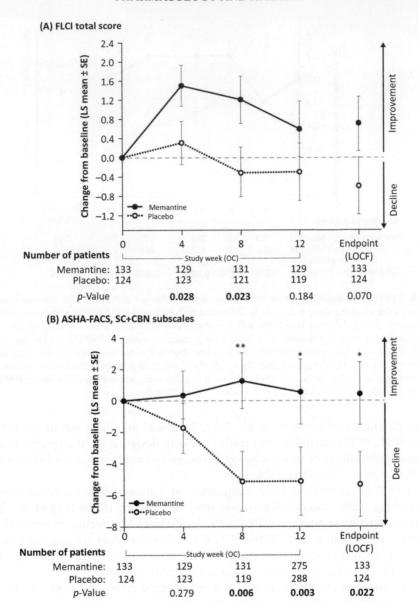

Figure 5. The effect of memantine on functional communication in patients with moderate Alzheimer's disease (Saxton et al., 2012). (A) Compared with placebo, memantine did not significantly improve functional communication at study endpoint (12 weeks, OC or LOCF), as assessed using the FLCI (score range 0–87), although the effect was significantly in favor of memantine at Weeks 4 and 8 (OC). (B) Memantine treatment significantly improved functional communication compared with placebo at study endpoint (LOCF) and Weeks 8 and 12 (OC), based on an assessment of caregivers, using the ASHA-FACS subscales of Social Communication and Communication of Basic Needs (score range 0–196). ASHA-FACS = American Speech-Language-Hearing Association Functional Assessment of Communication Skills for Adults scale; FLCI = Functional Linguistics Communication Inventory; LOCF = last observation carried forward; LS = least squares; OC = observed cases; SE = standard error. *$p < .05$; **$p < .01$; bold p-values indicate those attaining statistical significance. Reprinted with permission from IOS Press B.V. and Dr Judith Saxton. Figure originally published in *Journal of Alzheimer's Disease 28* (2008), 109–118.

treatment differences across the entire trial showed that patients taking memantine performed significantly better than those who received placebo ($p = .021$) (Saxton et al., 2012). In addition, caregivers of memantine-treated patients reported significantly better patient communication, compared with caregivers of placebo-treated patients, on the combined ASHA-FACS subscales at Week 8 (LOCF, $p = .008$ OC, $p = .006$) and endpoint (LOCF: $p = .022$; OC: $p = .033$) (see Figure 5B) (Saxton et al., 2012). These results of prospectively defined outcomes are in agreement with the *post hoc* analyses summarised above, in which the benefits of memantine on language and communication were observed on both objective measures of patient performance and subjective caregivers' impressions. The combined evidence of treatment differences detectable by both physicians and caregivers suggests that the effects of memantine on language in patients with AD are clinically relevant.

An open-label study, conducted in Germany and Austria, was designed to assess the efficacy of memantine treatment on measures of cognition and communication in patients with moderate-to-severe AD (MMSE 3–20) (Schulz et al., 2011). The primary efficacy parameter was the score change on the *Consortium to Establish a Registry for Alzheimer's Disease–Neuropsychological Battery* (CERAD–NP); secondary parameters included the FLCI and the semantic and phonemic *verbal fluency test*s. After 12 weeks of open-label memantine treatment, a significant improvement over baseline (mean ± standard deviation) was observed on the FLCI (4.4 ± 6.8; $p < .001$), with significant benefits being observed as early as Week 4 and largely maintained after a 4-week washout period (Schulz et al., 2011). Significant improvements over baseline were also observed on both the semantic (0.8 ± 3.0; $p < .01$) and the phonemic (1.2 ± 2.8; $p < .001$) *verbal fluency tests* (Schulz et al., 2011).

One additional trial, a single-group, open-label imaging study designed to assess changes in brain volume in memantine-treated patients with moderate AD (MEM-MD-15), also utilised cognitive measures as secondary outcomes, including several measures of language and communication (Weiner et al., 2011). In this trial, memantine was associated with significant improvement over baseline on the *Boston Naming Test*; however, semantic fluency and phonemic fluency showed no significant differences compared with baseline (see Table 1) (Saxton et al., 2012).

Aphasia due to other conditions

Although the efficacy of memantine has been primarily investigated in patients with AD, it also has been assessed in smaller studies involving patients with deficits in language and communication due to other conditions (see Table 2).

In a 52-week, open-label, placebo-controlled study involving patients with Parkinson's disease complicated with dementia, memantine-treated patients ($n = 32$) remained relatively stable on the phonemic *verbal fluency test*, while those treated with placebo ($n = 30$) demonstrated a significant decline from baseline. The difference between groups on this measure was significantly in favour of memantine at Week 24, as well as at Week 52 in a subset of patients with high homocysteine levels; no differences between groups were observed on the ADAS–cog at Week 52 (Litvinenko et al., 2010). In a 26-week open-label study of memantine in 43 patients with frontotemporal lobe degeneration (Boxer et al., 2009) memantine-treated patients with non-fluent progressive aphasia ($n = 9$) remained stable on the ADAS–cog after 26 weeks, patients with frontotemporal dementia

TABLE 2

Memantine treatment and language-related performance in non-Alzheimer's trials

Condition/study	Design, duration, size	Treatment	Language-related efficacy parameters	Memantine effect
Parkinson's Disease Dementia (Litvinenko et al., 2010) NCT not available	OL, placebo-controlled 52 weeks N = 62 PBO: 30 MEM: 32	MEM, 20 mg/d PBO	ADAS–cog D–KEFS—VFT FAB	Week 24 vs. PBO, all patients: VFT: $p < .05$ Week 52 vs. PBO, high homocysteine patients: VFT: $p < .05$ FAB: speech activity (verbal associations), $p = .02$
Frontotemporal Lobe Degeneration (Boxer et al., 2009) (FTD, Semantic Dementia, Non-fluent Progressive Aphasia) NCT00187525	OL 26 weeks N = 43 FTD: 21; Semantic Dementia: 13; Non-fluent Progressive Aphasia: 9	MEM, 20 mg/d (10 mg BID)	ADAS–cog	No significant between-group differences or significant improvements over baseline Patients with Progressive Aphasia remained relatively constant Significant decline in patients with Semantic Dementia ($p = .001$)
Frontotemporal Lobar Degeneration (Boxer et al., 2009) (bv FTD and Semantic Dementia) NCT00545974	RDBPC 26 weeks N = 81 bv FTD: n = 64 PBO: 33 MEM: 31 Semantic Dementia: n = 17 PBO: 9 MEM: 8	MEM, 20 mg/d (10 mg BID) PBO	VFT: phonemic VFT: semantic BNT	No significant difference between groups on VFT phonemic ($p = .75$) or VFT semantic ($p = .72$) MEM treatment was associated with a significant decline on BNT ($p = .004$)
Multiple Sclerosis (Lovera et al., 2010) NCT00300716	RDBPC 16 weeks N = 126 PBO: 68 MEM: 58	MEM, 20 mg/d (10 mg BID) PBO	COWAT	MEM treatment had no effect on any clinical measure

(Continued)

TABLE 2
(Continued)

Condition/study	Design, duration, size	Treatment	Language-related efficacy parameters	Memantine effect
Primary Progressive Aphasia (mild to moderate severity) (Johnson et al., 2010) NCT not available	RDBPC crossover 26 weeks treatment; 6 weeks down-titration/washout; 26 weeks crossover treatment $N = 18$	MEM, 20 mg/d (10 mg BID) PBO	WAB–AQ (others not specified)	No significant differences between MEM and PBO treatments, but a "trend" for decreased decline on the WAB–AQ observed with MEM
Chronic Post-stroke Aphasia (Berthier et al., 2009) NCT00640198	RDBPC (24 weeks) + OL extension (24 weeks) RDBPC: $N = 28$ PBO: 14 MEM: 14	RDBPC: MEM, 20 mg/d ± CIAT PBO ± CIAT OL: MEM	WAB–AQ CAL	RDBPC: Week 16 assessment: MEM was associated with a significant improvement over PBO on WAB–AQ total ($p = .002$) and the Naming subtest ($p = .015$)
	Weeks 1–16: MEM vs. PBO			Week 18 assessment: MEM + CIAT was associated with a significant improvement over PBO + CIAT on WAB–AQ total
	Weeks 17–18: MEM + CIAT vs. PBO + CIAT			($p < .001$) (and subtests of spontaneous speech, auditory comprehension and naming) and CAL ($p = .04$)
	Weeks 19–20: MEM vs. PBO			Addition of CIAT improved WAB–AQ and CAL scores in both groups, but the effect in the MEM group was stronger
	Weeks 21–24: MEM vs. PBO (washout)			OL:
	OL extension (Weeks 25–48): $N = 27$ PBO/MEM: 13 MEM/MEM: 14			Benefits persisted in MEM-treated patients; PBO-treated patients who switched to MEM improved significantly ($p = .02$)

(Continued)

TABLE 2
(Continued)

Condition/study	Design, duration, size	Treatment	Language-related efficacy parameters	Memantine effect
Women at Risk of Dementia (Wroolie et al., 2009) NCT00242632	OL 26 weeks of treatment + 26 weeks of follow-up N = 22	MEM, 20 mg/d	BNT VFT	MEM was associated with both positive and negative effects on language abilities; the negative effects were reversed after treatment discontinuation

ADAS–cog = Alzheimer's Disease Assessment Scale—cognitive subscale; BID = twice-daily dosing; bv = behavioural variant; CAL = Communicative Activity Log; BNT = Boston Naming Test; CIAT = constraint-induced aphasia therapy; COWAT = Controlled Oral Word Association Test; D–KEFS = Delis-Kaplan Executive Function System; FAB = Frontal Assessment Battery; FDG–PET = fluorodeoxyglucose—positron emission tomography; FTD = frontotemporal dementia; MEM = memantine; NCT = National Clinical Trial registration number; OL = open label; PBO = placebo; RDBPC = randomised double-blind placebo-controlled; VFT = Verbal Fluency Test; WAB–AQ = Western Aphasia Battery–Aphasia Quotient.

($n = 21$) demonstrated a slight, non-significant decline and patients with semantic dementia ($n = 13$) showed a significant within-group decline from baseline; however, there were no placebo-treated patients for comparison in any of the groups. A more recent, randomised, double-blind, placebo-controlled trial showed no advantage of memantine in patients with frontotemporal lobar degeneration (behavioural variant, $n = 64$; semantic dementia, $n = 17$) on primary endpoints of behaviour or global condition, and there was a significant, negative effect (worsening) in patients treated with memantine on the *Boston Naming Test*; no difference was seen on either *verbal fluency test* measure (Boxer et al., 2013). There were also numerically more cognitive adverse events (confusion, memory loss, language disorders) in the memantine group in this study. In patients with multiple sclerosis (Lovera et al., 2010), a 16-week randomised trial ($N = 126$) did not show any benefits of memantine over placebo on any outcome measure.

In a pilot randomised, crossover, double-bind, placebo-controlled trial of patients with mild-to-moderate primary progressive aphasia ($N = 18$) (Johnson et al., 2010), 26 weeks of memantine treatment was associated with a smaller decline on the *Western Aphasia Battery—Aphasia Quotient* (Kertesz, 1982) compared with placebo treatment, although this difference did not reach significance. Similarly, a 24-week, randomised, double-blind, placebo-controlled trial of memantine in patients with chronic post-stroke aphasia ($N = 28$) demonstrated a significant improvement over placebo on two measures of aphasia (*Western Aphasia Battery—Aphasia Quotient and Communicative Activity Log*), which was augmented when combined with constraint-induced aphasia therapy (Berthier et al., 2009). In this study, the benefits of memantine treatment persisted throughout a subsequent 24-week open-label phase, and patients treated with placebo improved significantly upon switching to memantine (Berthier et al., 2009). Finally, in a study of post-menopausal women at risk of cognitive decline due to possession of the apoE-ϵ4 gene, personal or family history of a mood disorder, hypothyroidism or family history of AD ($N = 22$), an improvement that approached statistical significance ($p = .077$) on the Verbal Fluency Category Switching of the *Delis–Kaplan Executive Function System* was observed after 6 months of open-label memantine treatment, and a significant improvement over baseline on the *Boston Naming Test* ($p = .025$) was observed 6 months after treatment discontinuation (Wroolie et al., 2009).

DISCUSSION AND CONCLUSIONS

Communication-related problems in patients with AD are among the most common issues cited by caregivers as a source of burden (Kinney & Stephens, 1989; Ripich, 1994; Savundranayagam, Hummert, & Montgomery, 2005). Language impairment is also a core feature of two variants of frontotemporal dementia, semantic dementia (involving loss of verbal comprehension and object knowledge) and progressive non-fluent aphasia (hesitant, non-fluent speech) (Cardarelli, Kertesz, & Knebl, 2010). In addition to making information exchange more challenging, communication impairment may also trigger problem behaviours, such as agitation and aggression in patients with AD, which have been shown to further increase emotional strain and demand for caregiver time (Savundranayagam et al., 2005; Woodward, 2013). In patients with stroke-induced aphasia, the production of speech itself is a source of anxiety, stress and labour, such that the anticipation of error may exacerbate or contribute to the primary communication difficulty (Cahana-Amitay et al., 2011).

Yet, despite the prevalence and importance of symptoms related to language and communication in these and other conditions, very few studies have investigated the use of pharmacological agents for their alleviation (Cahana-Amitay et al., 2011; Saxton et al., 2012).

Memantine, a moderate-affinity, uncompetitive antagonist of NMDA glutamate receptors (Parsons et al., 2007) approved for the treatment of moderate-to-severe AD (Forest Pharmaceuticals, 2007; McShane et al., 2006), has been demonstrated to provide modest benefits on language in multiple studies of patients with AD, using several different outcome measures (Grossberg et al., 2013; Saxton et al., 2012; Schmitt et al., 2006; Schulz et al., 2011; Tocco et al., 2008; Tocco & Graham, 2010; Weiner et al., 2011). Although it is difficult to isolate benefits on language per se from benefits on attention and memory (see below), the improvements observed using both objective measurements (Grossberg et al., 2013; Saxton et al., 2012; Schmitt et al., 2006; Schulz et al., 2011) and caregivers' impressions (Saxton et al., 2012) suggest that memantine provides a positive effect on communication. Memantine has also been shown to decrease agitation and aggression in clinical trials (Gauthier, Loft, & Cummings, 2008). Since it has been hypothesised that such problem behaviours may be partially caused by the inability of patients to effectively communicate (Savundranayagam et al., 2005; Woodward, 2013), it is interesting to speculate whether the effects of memantine on agitation and aggression occur directly, through the pharmacological modulation of neural pathways that regulate these behaviours, or indirectly, by improving communication.

The effects of memantine on language and communication abilities in patients with conditions other than AD have thus far been mixed: some evidence for language improvements exists for patients with Parkinson's disease dementia (Litvinenko et al., 2010) and aphasia due to stroke (Berthier et al., 2009), but not for patients with frontotemporal dementia (Boxer et al., 2009, 2013; Chow et al., 2011, 2013), primary progressive aphasia (Johnson et al., 2010) or multiple sclerosis (Lovera et al., 2010), while the effects of memantine on communication-related measures in postmenopausal women at risk for dementia were mixed (Wroolie et al., 2009). It is unclear to what extent these disparities reflect differences in underlying pathology between the various populations, differences in trial design and assessment or simply a lack of statistical power in studies with small sample sizes.

Our analysis is limited by a number of factors. In many of the conditions studied, language deficits are secondary to impairment in memory or executive abilities, so very few of the outcome measures used in the studies were specifically designed to assess functional communication per se. Even in populations that were primarily impaired in language domains (semantic dementia, primary progressive aphasia), the outcome measures chosen typically were insufficient to measure these deficits. For example, the authors of an imaging study in patients with frontotemporal dementia point out in their discussion that "despite our sample consisting mainly of semantic dementia, we did not test participants using aphasia test scores beyond the semantic fluency item on the *Frontal Assessment Battery*, and so the effect of memantine on language has not been examined" (Chow et al., 2013). To complicate matters further, many of the trials listed were small and limited in statistical power, as discussed above. Despite these limitations, however, the collective evidence suggests a potential for improvements in language abilities with memantine treatment, across a wide variety of conditions. Therefore, conducting a large-scale clinical trial of memantine across patients with language impairments due to multiple aetiologies may be useful. Although the exact composition of the trial population and the assessment tools utilised would need to be established, it would be of interest to determine whether memantine exerts a common effect on neuronal pathways related to communication in general.

REFERENCES

Ahmed, S., de Jager, C. A., Haigh, A. M., & Garrard, P. (2012). Logopenic aphasia in Alzheimer's disease: Clinical variant or clinical feature? *Journal of Neurology, Neurosurgery & Psychiatry, 83*(11), 1056–1062.

Bakchine, S., & Loft, H. (2008). Memantine treatment in patients with mild to moderate Alzheimer's disease: Results of a randomised, double-blind, placebo-controlled 6-month study. *Journal of Alzheimer's Disease, 13*(1), 97–107.

Bayles, K. A., & Tomoeda, C. K. (1994). *Functional linguistic communication inventory*. Tucson, AZ: Canyonlands Publishing.

Bayles, K. A., Tomoeda, C. K., Cruz, R. F., & Mahendra, N. (2000). Communication abilities of individuals with late-stage Alzheimer disease. *Alzheimer Disease and Associated Disorders, 14*(3), 176–181.

Berthier, M. L. (2005). Poststroke aphasia: Epidemiology, pathophysiology and treatment. *Drugs Aging, 22*(2), 163–182.

Berthier, M. L., Green, C., Lara, J. P., Higueras, C., Barbancho, M. A., Davila, G., & Pulvermuller, F. (2009). Memantine and constraint-induced aphasia therapy in chronic poststroke aphasia. *Annals of Neurology, 65*(5), 577–585.

Boxer, A. L., Knopman, D. S., Kaufer, D. I., Grossman, M., Onyike, C., Graf-Radford, N., . . . Miller, B. L. (2013). Memantine in patients with frontotemporal lobar degeneration: A multicentre, randomised, double-blind, placebo-controlled trial. *Lancet Neurology, 12*(2), 149–156.

Boxer, A. L., Lipton, A. M., Womack, K., Merrilees, J., Neuhaus, J., Pavlic, D., . . . Miller, B. L. (2009). An open-label study of memantine treatment in 3 subtypes of frontotemporal lobar degeneration. *Alzheimer Disease and Associated Disorders, 23*(3), 211–217.

Cahana-Amitay, D., Albert, M. L., Pyun, S. B., Westwood, A., Jenkins, T., Wolford, S., & Finley, M. (2011). Language as a stressor in aphasia. *aphasiology, 25*(2), 593–614.

Cardarelli, R., Kertesz, A., & Knebl, J. A. (2010). Frontotemporal dementia: A review for primary care physicians. *American Family Physician, 82*(11), 1372–1377.

Chez, M. G., Burton, Q., Dowling, T., Chang, M., Khanna, P., & Kramer, C. (2007). Memantine as adjunctive therapy in children diagnosed with autistic spectrum disorders: An observation of initial clinical response and maintenance tolerability. *Journal of Child Neurology, 22*(5), 574–579.

Choudhury, P. R., Lahiri, S., & Rajamma, U. (2012). Glutamate mediated signaling in the pathophysiology of autism spectrum disorders. *Pharmacology Biochemistry and Behavior, 100*(4), 841–849.

Chow, T. W., Fam, D., Graff-Guerrero, A., Verhoeff, N. P., Tang-Wai, D. F., Masellis, M., . . . Pollock, B. G. (2013). Fluorodeoxyglucose positron emission tomography in semantic dementia after 6 months of memantine: An open-label pilot study. *International Journal of Geriatric Psychiatry, 28*(3), 319–325.

Chow, T. W., Graff-Guerrero, A., Verhoeff, N. P., Binns, M. A., Tang-Wai, D. F., Freedman, M., . . . Pollock, B. G. (2011). Open-label study of the short-term effects of memantine on FDG-PET in frontotemporal dementia. *Neuropsychiatric Disease and Treatment, 7*, 415–424.

Emre, M., Mecocci, P., & Stender, K. (2008). Pooled analyses on cognitive effects of memantine in patients with moderate to severe Alzheimer's disease. *Journal of Alzheimer's Disease, 14*(2), 193–199.

Ferris, S., Ihl, R., Robert, P., Winblad, B., Gatz, G., Tennigkeit, F., & Gauthier, S. (2009a). Severe impairment battery language scale: A language-assessment tool for Alzheimer's disease patients. *Alzheimer's & Dementia, 5*(5), 375–379.

Ferris, S., Ihl, R., Robert, P., Winblad, B., Gatz, G., Tennigkeit, F., & Gauthier, S. (2009b). Treatment effects of memantine on language in moderate to severe Alzheimer's disease patients. *Alzheimer's & Dementia, 5*(5), 369–374.

Folstein, M. F., Folstein, S. E., & McHugh, P. R. (1975). Mini-mental state. A practical method for grading the cognitive state of patients for the clinician. *Journal of Psychiatric Research, 12*(3), 189–198.

Forest Pharmaceuticals Inc. (2007). *Namenda®: U.S. Prescribing Information*. St. Louis, MO: Forest Pharmaceuticals.

Forstl, H., & Kurz, A. (1999). Clinical features of Alzheimer's disease. *European Archives of Psychiatry and Clinical Neurosciences, 249*(6), 288–290.

Francis, P. T. (2009). Altered glutamate neurotransmission and behaviour in dementia: Evidence from studies of memantine. *Current Molecular Pharmacology, 2*(1), 77–82.

Frattali, C. M., Thompson, C. K., Holland, A. L., Wohl, C. B., & Ferketic, M. M. (1995). *Functional assessment of communication skills for adults (ASHA FACS).* Rockville, MD: American Speech-Language-Hearing Association.

Fromm, D., & Holland, A. (1989). Functional communication in Alzheimer's disease. *The Journal of Speech and Hearing Disorders, 54*(4), 535–540.

Galasko, D., Bennett, D., Sano, M., Ernesto, C., Thomas, R., Grundman, M., & Ferris, S. (1997). An inventory to assess activities of daily living for clinical trials in Alzheimer's disease. The Alzheimer's Disease Cooperative Study. *Alzheimer Disease and Associated Disorders, 11*(Suppl 2), S33–S39.

Galasko, D., Schmitt, F., Thomas, R., Jin, S., & Bennett, D. (2005). Detailed assessment of activities of daily living in moderate to severe Alzheimer's disease. *Journal of the International Neuropsychological Society, 11*(4), 446–453.

Gauthier, S., Loft, H., & Cummings, J. (2008). Improvement in behavioural symptoms in patients with moderate to severe Alzheimer's disease by memantine: A pooled data analysis. *International Journal of Geriatric Psychiatry, 23*(5), 537–545.

Ghezzi, A., Goretti, B., Portaccio, E., Roscio, M., & Amato, M. P. (2010). Cognitive impairment in pediatric multiple sclerosis. *Neurological Sciences, 31*(Suppl 2), S215–S218.

Gorno-Tempini, M. L., Hillis, A. E., Weintraub, S., Kertesz, A., Mendez, M., Cappa, S. F., . . . Grossman, M. (2011). Classification of primary progressive aphasia and its variants. *Neurology, 76*(11), 1006–1014.

Grossberg, G. T., Manes, F., Allegri, R. F., Gutierrez-Robledo, L. M., Gloger, S., Xie, L., . . . Graham, S. (2013). The safety, tolerability, and efficacy of once-daily memantine (28 mg): A multinational, ran-domized, double-blind, placebo-controlled trial in patients with moderate-tosevere Alzheimer's disease taking cholinesterase inhibitors. *CNS Drugs, 27*(6), 469–478.

Honig, L. S., & Mayeux, R. (2001). Natural history of Alzheimer's disease. *Aging (Milano), 13*(3), 171–182.

Isaacs, B., & Kennie, A. T. (1973). The Set test as an aid to the detection of dementia in old people. *The British Journal of Psychiatry, 123*(575), 467–470.

Johnson, N. A., Rademaker, A., Weintraub, S., Gitelman, D., Wienecke, C., & Mesulam, M. (2010). Pilot trial of memantine in primary progressive aphasia. *Alzheimer Disease and Associated Disorders, 24*(3), 308.

Kertesz, A. (1982). *Western aphasia battery (WAB).* San Antonio, TX: The Psychological Corporation.

Kinney, J. M., & Stephens, M. A. (1989). Caregiving hassles scale: Assessing the daily hassles of caring for a family member with dementia. *Gerontologist, 29*(3), 328–332.

Kitamura, S., Honma, A., Nakamura, Y., & Yoshimura, I. (2011). Late phase II study of memantine hydrochloride, a new NMDA receptor antagonist, in patients with moderate to severe Alzheimer's disease: Efficacy, safety and recommended dose. *Japanese Journal of Geriatric Psychiatry, 22*, 300–311.

Litvinenko, I. V., Odinak, M. M., Mogil'naya, V. I., & Perstnev, S. V. (2010). Use of memantine (akati-nol) for the correction of cognitive impairments in Parkinson's disease complicated by dementia. *Neuroscience and Behavioral Physiology, 40*(2), 149–155.

Lovera, J. F., Frohman, E., Brown, T. R., Bandari, D., Nguyen, L., Yadav, V., . . . Bourdette, D. (2010). Memantine for cognitive impairment in multiple sclerosis: A randomized placebo-controlled trial. *Multiple Sclerosis, 16*(6), 715–723.

McShane, R., Areosa Sastre, A., & Minakaran, N. (2006). Memantine for dementia. *Cochrane Database of Systematic Reviews*, (2), CD003154.

Mecocci, P., Bladstrom, A., & Stender, K. (2009). Effects of memantine on cognition in patients with moderate to severe Alzheimer's disease: Post-hoc analyses of ADAS-cog and SIB total and single-item scores from six randomized, double-blind, placebo-controlled studies. *International Journal of Geriatric Psychiatry, 24*(5), 532–538.

Mesulam, M. M. (2003). Primary progressive aphasia–A language-based dementia. *The New England Journal of Medicine, 349*(16), 1535–1542.

Morris, J. C., Heyman, A., Mohs, R. C., Hughes, J. P., van Belle, G., Fillenbaum, G., . . . Clark, C. (1989). The Consortium to Establish a Registry for Alzheimer's Disease (CERAD). Part I. Clinical and neuropsychological assessment of Alzheimer's disease. *Neurology, 39*(9), 1159–1165.

Ocklenburg, S., Arning, L., Hahn, C., Gerding, W. M., Epplen, J. T., Gunturkun, O., & Beste, C. (2011). Variation in the NMDA receptor 2B subunit gene GRIN2B is associated with differential language lateralization. *Behavioural Brain Research, 225*(1), 284–289.

Panisset, M., Roudier, M., Saxton, J., & Boller, F. (1994). Severe impairment battery. A neuropsychological test for severely demented patients. *Archives of Neurology, 51*(1), 41–45.

Parsons, C. G., Danysz, W., & Quack, G. (1999). Memantine is a clinically well tolerated *N*-methyl-D-aspartate (NMDA) receptor antagonist—A review of preclinical data. *Neuropharmacology, 38*(6), 735–767.

Parsons, C. G., Stoffler, A., & Danysz, W. (2007). Memantine: A NMDA receptor antagonist that improves memory by restoration of homeostasis in the glutamatergic system—Too little activation is bad, too much is even worse. *Neuropharmacology, 53*(6), 699–723.

Peskind, E. R., Potkin, S. G., Pomara, N., Ott, B. R., Graham, S. M., Olin, J. T., & McDonald, S. (2006). Memantine treatment in mild to moderate Alzheimer disease: A 24-week randomized, controlled trial. *The American Journal of Geriatric Psychiatry, 14*(8), 704–715.

Pomara, N., Ott, B. R., Peskind, E., & Resnick, E. M. (2007). Memantine treatment of cognitive symptoms in mild to moderate Alzheimer disease: Secondary analyses from a placebo-controlled randomized trial. *Alzheimer Disease and Associated Disorders, 21*(1), 60–64.

Porsteinsson, A. P., Grossberg, G. T., Mintzer, J., & Olin, J. T. (2008). Memantine treatment in patients with mild to moderate Alzheimer's disease already receiving a cholinesterase inhibitor: A randomized, double-blind, placebo-controlled trial. *Current Alzheimer Research, 5*(1), 83–89.

Portugal Mda, G., Marinho, V., & Laks, J. (2011). Pharmacological treatment of frontotemporal lobar degeneration: Systematic review. *Revista Brasileira de Psiquiatria, 33*(1), 81–90.

Pulvermüller, F., & Berthier, M. L. (2008). Aphasia therapy on a neuroscience basis. *Aphasiology, 22*(6), 563–599.

Reilly, J., Rodriguez, A. D., Lamy, M., & Neils-Strunjas, J. (2010). Cognition, language, and clinical pathological features of non-Alzheimer's dementias: An overview. *Journal of Communication Disorders, 43*(5), 438–452.

Reisberg, B., Doody, R., Stoffler, A., Schmitt, F., Ferris, S., & Mobius, H. J. (2003). Memantine in moderate-to-severe Alzheimer's disease. *The New England Journal of Medicine, 348*(14), 1333–1341.

Ripich, D. N. (1994). Functional communication with AD patients: A caregiver training program. *Alzheimer Disease and Associated Disorders, 8*(Suppl 3), 95–109.

Rosen, W. G., Mohs, R. C., & Davis, K. L. (1984). A new rating scale for Alzheimer's disease. *The American Journal of Psychiatry, 141*(11), 1356–1364.

Sani, G., Serra, G., Kotzalidis, G. D., Romano, S., Tamorri, S. M., Manfredi, G., . . . Girardi, P. (2012). The role of memantine in the treatment of psychiatric disorders other than the dementias: A review of current preclinical and clinical evidence. *CNS Drugs, 26*(8), 663–690.

Saur, D., & Hartwigsen, G. (2012). Neurobiology of language recovery after stroke: Lessons from neuroimaging studies. *Archives of Physical Medicine and Rehabilitation, 93*(1 Suppl), S15–S25.

Savundranayagam, M. Y., Hummert, M. L., & Montgomery, R. J. (2005). Investigating the effects of communication problems on caregiver burden. *The Journals of Gerontology Series B: Psychological Sciences and Social Sciences, 60*(1), S48–55.

Saxton, J., Hofbauer, R. K., Woodward, M., Gilchrist, N. L., Potocnik, F., Hsu, H. A., . . . Perhach, J. L. (2012). Memantine and functional communication in Alzheimer's disease: Results of a 12-week, international, randomized clinical trial. *Journal of Alzheimer's Disease, 28*(1), 109–118.

Schmitt, F. A., Ashford, W., Ernesto, C., Saxton, J., Schneider, L. S., Clark, C. M., . . . Thal, L. J. (1997). The severe impairment battery: Concurrent validity and the assessment of longitudinal change in Alzheimer's disease. The Alzheimer's Disease Cooperative Study. *Alzheimer Disease and Associated Disorders, 11*(Suppl 2), S51–S56.

Schmitt, F. A., van Dyck, C. H., Wichems, C. H., & Olin, J. T. (2006). Cognitive response to memantine in moderate to severe Alzheimer disease patients already receiving donepezil: An exploratory reanalysis. *Alzheimer Disease and Associated Disorders, 20*(4), 255–262.

Schulz, J. B., Rainer, M., Klunemann, H. H., Kurz, A., Wolf, S., Sternberg, K., & Tennigkeit, F. (2011). Sustained effects of once-daily memantine treatment on cognition and functional communication skills in patients with moderate to severe Alzheimer's disease: Results of a 16-week open-label trial. *Journal of Alzheimer's Disease, 25*(3), 463–475.

Tariot, P. N., Farlow, M. R., Grossberg, G. T., Graham, S. M., McDonald, S., & Gergel, I. (2004). Memantine treatment in patients with moderate to severe Alzheimer disease already receiving donepezil: A randomized controlled trial. *JAMA, 291*(3), 317–324.

Tocco, M. T., & Graham, S. M. (2010). Effects of memantine treatment on language abilities and functional communication in patients with moderate to severe Alzheimer's disease: A review of data [abstract]. *Alzheimer's & Dementia, 6*(Suppl. 4), S304.

Tocco, M. T., Saxton, J., Tariot, P., Hofbauer, R. K., Resnick, E. M., & Graham, S. M. (2008). Effects of memantine on language and functional communication in patients with moderate to severe Alzheimer's disease receiving stable doses of donepezil [abstract]. *Neurology, 70*(Suppl. 1), A99.

van der Kam, P., Mol, F., & Wimmers, M. (1971). *Beoordelingsschaal voor oudere patienten (BOP)*. Deventer: Van Loghum Slaterus.

van Dyck, C. H., Tariot, P. N., Meyers, B., & Resnick, E. M. (2007). A 24-week randomized, controlled trial of memantine in patients with moderate-to-severe Alzheimer disease. *Alzheimer Disease and Associated Disorders, 21*(2), 136–143.

Verma, M., & Howard, R. J. (2012). Semantic memory and language dysfunction in early Alzheimer's disease: A review. *International Journal of Geriatric Psychiatry, 27*(12), 1209–1217.

Weiner, M. W., Sadowsky, C., Saxton, J., Hofbauer, R. K., Graham, S. M., Yu, S. Y., . . . Perhach, J. L. (2011). Magnetic resonance imaging and neuropsychological results from a trial of memantine in Alzheimer's disease. *Alzheimer's & Dementia, 7*(4), 425–435.

Woodward, M. (2013). Aspects of communication in Alzheimer's disease: Clinical features and treatment options. *International Psychogeriatrics, 25*(6), 877–885.

Wroolie, T. E., Kenna, H. A., Williams, K. E., Powers, B. N., Holcomb, M., Lazzeroni, L., & Rasgon, N. L. (2009). Cognitive effects of memantine in postmenopausal women at risk of dementia: A pilot study. *Acta Neurologica Scandinavica, 119*(3), 172–179.

Zec, R. F., Landreth, E. S., Fritz, S., Grames, E., Hasara, A., Fraizer, W., . . . Manyam, B. (1999). A comparison of phonemic, semantic, and alternating word fluency in Parkinson's disease. *Archives of Clinical Neuropsychology, 14*(3), 255–264.

Index

Note: Page numbers in **bold** type refer to **figures**
Page numbers in *italic* type refer to *tables*

Printed and bound by CPI Group (UK) Ltd, Croydon, CR0 4YY

24/10/2024

01778294-0003